Interprofessional Education

Interprofessional Education

Making It Happen

Edited by

Patricia Bluteau and Ann Jackson

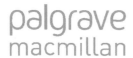

First published 2009 by
PALGRAVE MACMILLAN

Palgrave Macmillan in the UK is an imprint of Macmillan Publishers Limited, registered in England, company number 785998, of Houndmills, Basingstoke, Hampshire RG21 6XS.

Palgrave Macmillan in the US is a division of St Martin's Press LLC, 175 Fifth Avenue, New York, NY 10010.

Palgrave Macmillan is the global academic imprint of the above companies and has companies and representatives throughout the world.

Palgrave® and Macmillan® are registered trademarks in the United States, the United Kingdom, Europe and other countries.

ISBN 978–0–230–57447–2

This book is printed on paper suitable for recycling and made from fully managed and sustained forest sources. Logging, pulping and manufacturing processes are expected to conform to the environmental regulations of the country of origin.

A catalogue record for this book is available from the British Library.

10   9   8   7   6   5   4   3   2   1
18   17   16   15   14   13   12   11   10   09

Printed in China

Contents

Foreword

I am not aware of any one book that covers the terrain of this volume. For me it had some of the excitement of discovering the power of satellite mapping – laid out before me was a more realistic representation than I had ever previously seen of familiar ground: I was able both to scan across the breadth of Interprofessional Education (IPE) and to explore in greater depth than was previously possible.

The historical context is laid out with unparalleled authority by Hugh Barr; this is not simply a matter of great interest for all who are interested in the field, it is also an essential understanding for those who wish to learn from what has been tried in the past. That policy initiatives have met with mixed success should come as no surprise to practitioners, but the expertise and experience of the editorial team is evident in the way that clear pathways emerge through the maze in Pat Bluteau and Ann Jackson's exposition of how IPE can make real contributions to the all-important interprofessional working.

With the work of the Joint Evaluation Team early in this century, the important question moved on from whether IPE is effective to 'How, and under what circumstances is interprofessional education effective?' Helen Langton's contribution to this book is to set out very clearly the contribution of academia (potential and realised) to IPE. Collaboration is at the heart of interprofessional learning and practice, so it is helpful to learn from Frances Gordon about the potential for collaboration between universities. The construction of this volume is beautifully logical in that Part II explores for practitioners the practical approaches which have a theoretical rationale in terms of the subject overview in Part I. Thus Jackson and Bluteau bring to life the potential for university contributions so carefully developed by Langton.

Unlike many books written by enthusiasts in contended areas, there is no attempt here to avoid discussion of tricky questions about the evidence for effectiveness. Part III is dedicated to evaluation, starting with the well-known work on readiness for interprofessional learning. Karen Mattick and John Bligh have seized the opportunity here to create a chapter which should be required reading for all concerned with evaluation in clinical education: they not only trace the development of a key instrument in IPL, demonstrating the rigour that it required for such development, but they also manage to show the impact of developing this instrument in taking forward the study of IPL. Sarah Hean's chapter on stereotypes is of similar importance. For me this chapter acts as a reflective pause: familiar concepts re-examined in context and afforded new meaning. Those with a research bent will again glean much of practical importance in Suzanne Lindqvist's account of questionnaire development in researching IPL.

The real world application of IPE is emphasised by Jackson and Bluteau's grasp of the important aspects of operationalising learning in order for practice in health and social care to improve and with it the quality of the patient experience. Leaders and managers have to do more than pay lip-service if the gains of having struggled to overcome the numerous obstacles to effective IPL are not to be eroded by unsupportive workplace environments. Who better to round off the authoritative overview than Marilyn Hammick and Liz Anderson, both of whom have been central to IPL projects and steering over the past decade in the UK.

The map is before you. What are you going to do with it?

ED PEILE
Professor Emeritus of Clinical Education
Warwick Medical School

Preface

A few years ago when Interprofessional Education (IPE) became more mainstream and a requirement of most health and social care curricula, we found ourselves searching for guidance, information and support on developing, implementing, delivering and evaluating IPE both in academic and practice settings. We wanted to understand the historical development in order to contextualise IPE both for ourselves and our students. This was all available but not in one place. The Centre for the Advancement of Interprofessional Education (CAIPE) proved invaluable in the early days but as we began to develop IPE opportunities in both settings we were met with a myriad of challenges and obstacles. Naively, we had not expected the degree of resistance, misunderstanding and professional fears associated with collaborative endeavours. In those early days little had been written about these challenges, although literature is now emerging which highlights the difficulty of changing cultures and beliefs.

We deliberately invited the authors featured in this book as they were able to offer particular expertise in key areas for professionals involved in developing, delivering and evaluating IPE. As a consequence each chapter is written in each author's unique style, and can be used in isolation to develop the understanding of each key area, or can be used to as a toolkit to facilitate IPE initiatives.

We hope that many people will enjoy this book, find it useful and be engaged by the material found within.

PAT & ANN

Note to readers: We are aware that across health and social care professional groups a variety of terms are used to describe the person receiving care. In this book such a person has been described as a patient, client or service user. We wish it to be known that whilst we use a range of nouns to describe such a person we in no way wish to disempower an individual.

Acknowledgements

They say that life is what happens when you are busy making other plans. This couldn't be truer for not only the editors, but also several of the contributors to this book. Personal tragedies and triumphs have simultaneously occurred alongside normal academic and home demands delaying the completion of this book. We would like to acknowledge the contributors who have, in many cases, patiently accommodated these demands and delays; to them we offer a big thank you.

We deeply value the support given by our families: André and Joshua, John and Steven. In addition, we would also like to thank the individuals who supported our contributing authors, and most importantly each other, as we shared the journey.

The authors and publishers wish to thank the following for permission to use copyright material: Sheffield University for use of Tables 4.1–4.4; Coventry University for the screenshots from the *Interprofessional Learning Pathway* website in Chapter 6 and the appendices; Wiley-Blackwell for Table 8.1 from Carpenter, J. (1995b). Interprofessional education for medical and nursing students: Evaluation of a programme. *Medical Education*, 29 (4), 265–272.; Table 8.2 from Mandy, A., C. Milton, and P. Mandy. (2004). Professional stereotyping and interprofessional education. *Learning in Health and Social Care*, 3, 154–170 and Figure 8.1 from Hean, S., J. Macleod Clark, K. Adams, and D. Humphris. (2006a). Will opposites attract? Similarities and differences in students' perceptions of the stereotype profiles of other health and social care professional groups. *Journal of Interprofessional Care*, 20 (2), 162–181; John Carpenter for Table 8.3 from Carpenter, J., D. Barnes, and C. Dickinson. (2003). Making a modern mental health care workforce: Evaluation of the Birmingham University Interprofessional Training Programme in Community Mental Health 1998–2002. Durham: Centre for Applied Social Studies, University of Durham; Warwick Medical School, Coventry University and South Warwickshire Primary Care Trust for the *Interprofessional Learning Week: Information Guide for Students* and the *Interprofessional Learning Week: Information Guide for Experts and Facilitators*; Coventry University and University of Warwick for *Interprofessional*

Learning Pathway Year 1 and *Facilitator Guide: Year 3*. Every effort has been made to trace the copyright holders, but if any have been inadvertently overlooked the publishers will be pleased to make the necessary arrangements at the first opportunity.

PAT BLUTEAU & ANN JACKSON

Notes on Contributors

Elizabeth Anderson. Senior Lecturer in Shared Learning in the Department of Medical and Social Care Education, University of Leicester, UK.

Hugh Barr. Professor Emeritus in Interprofessional Education, University of Westminster, London, UK.

John Bligh. Professor of Clinical Education and Vice Dean at the Peninsula Medical School, Exeter, UK.

Patricia Bluteau. Associate Director of Centre for Interprofessional e learning, School of Health and Social Sciences, Coventry University, UK.

Frances Gordon. Professor of Interprofessional Education, Head of Interprofessional and Multidisciplinary Learning and Director of the Centre for Interprofessional e learning (CIPeL), Sheffield Hallam University, Sheffield, UK.

Marilyn Hammick. Professor, Learning and Teaching consultant – Research and Evaluation, The Higher Education Academy, Health Sciences and Practice, London, UK.

Sarah Hean. Senior Lecturer – Research, The School of Health & Social Care Bournemouth University, UK.

Ann Jackson. Associate Professor Interprofessional Education, Institute of Clinical Education, Warwick Medical School, University of Warwick, UK.

Helen Langton. Professor and Dean, Faculty of Education, Health and Sciences, University of Derby, UK.

Suzanne Lindqvist. Centre Director and Lecturer in Interprofessional Practice, University of East Anglia, UK.

Karen Mattick. Senior Lecturer in Clinical Education, Peninsula College of Medicine and Dentistry, Exeter, UK.

Ed Peile. Professor Emeritus of Clinical Education, Warwick Medical School, University of Warwick, UK.

Part I

The Background to Interprofessional Education

This part is made up of four chapters. Internationally renowned authors offer a background to the development of interprofessional education (IPE). In Chapter 1, Hugh Barr, discusses the early beginning of IPE, the growth and development and key challenges along the way. In Chapter 2, Pat Bluteau and Ann Jackson build on this work, by looking back over time and highlighting some of the key challenges within education in achieving collaboration, whilst discussing the challenges to lecturers in higher education and the implications of shared learning.

In Chapter 3, Helen Langton moves on to concentrate on the ways in which interprofessional learning has developed in academic settings, reviewing a variety of models and methods of delivery in IPE. The chapter considers a range of models which include three distinct approaches which are driven in different ways – modular, learning outcomes and thematic. It also offers insight into the manner in which higher education institutions have introduced and modified their IPE strategy over time, in relation to their experiences which are offered to the reader.

In Chapter 4, Frances Gordon completes Part I of the book with an explanation of the development of the Combined Universities Interprofessional Learning Unit (CUILU) capability framework – developed specifically for practice based IPE.

While UK initiatives are drawn on, experiences internationally mirror those of the UK. These four chapters encourage the reader in both health and social care arenas to consider the background lessons learned. They also offer transferable experiences and frameworks that can be built into new or developed for existing programmes.

1

Interprofessional Education as an Emerging Concept

Hugh Barr

Introduction

Interprofessional education (IPE) in the UK originated in innumerable discrete 'initiatives' unbeknown to each other in diverse fields of practice. The Centre for the Advancement of Interprofessional Education (CAIPE) opened up channels for communication within and between those fields, complemented later by the Higher Education Academy. The World Health Organization (WHO) including UK initiatives in its global review, while the *Journal of Interprofessional Care*, launched in and for the UK, became the conduit for exchange between national and international developments.

The CAIPE defined IPE, enunciated principles, formulated outcomes and set standards in search of coherence, consensus and consistency, overtaken by a government-led agenda for 'common learning' initially to promote collaborative practice, but increasingly to develop a more flexible workforce to assist in modernising health and social care services. These twin objectives carried different implications for interprofessional content and learning methods, differences which remain ill-understood and ill-addressed.

Introducing Interprofessional Education

IPE began in the UK during the 1960s. Early 'initiatives' were invariably local, small-scale, isolated, ephemeral and work based in primary or community care. Their instigators were driven on the one hand by belief in teamworking as the means to respond more fully and more effectively to the needs of patients and clients,[1] on the other by growing awareness of the need to resolve tensions between professions practising in close proximity for the first time. Teamwork, as it became apparent, was no panacea. Opportunities had to be created where members could learn about each other's values, knowledge, skills, roles and responsibilities, and reconcile differences, either during team meetings or time out such as awaydays. Many of these initiatives were in primary care, others in fields such as learning disabilities, mental illness, elder care or palliative care where learning together often focused also on shared understanding and ownership of progressive models of care and joint action to implement them. Each initiative was learned by trial and error with few, if any, opportunities to compare experience within the same field, let alone across fields, but with uncanny similarities (Barr 2007a).

IPE in child protection started later. It was driven by reports from successive enquiries into the abuse and sometimes death of children from 1972 onwards (Hallett and Birchall 1992) calling for 'joint training' to improve communications and trust between professions variously responsible for their education, health and wellbeing. The emphasis was less on teamwork, more on networking, establishing machinery for effective collaboration between agencies as much as professions. Exchange of experience between IPE in child protection and in primary and community care was conspicuous by its absence for many years.

So long as IPE was work based, it remained largely hidden. If and when initiatives were recorded, reports were usually for local consumption, few surviving the passage of time or finding their way into publications. IPE was, however, also taking hold in universities and colleges where it was more visible. Most of those initiatives were at the post-registration stage, typically recruiting experienced practitioners from a range of professions on to part-time courses to enhance theoretical and evidence-based understanding of specialist practice with a particular patient group or in a particular field. Fewer were during pre-registration studies. Indeed, it is sometimes unclear from the sketchy reports surviving which of these were intra-professional, for example between branches of nursing or social work, and which were interprofessional as understood in this book. Some of the teachers pioneering these initiatives reported their experience within their respective fields through papers presented at conferences and in journals, less often between fields.

Much of the credit for drawing IPE initiatives together in the UK goes to the CAIPE[2] launched in 1987. CAIPE focused initially on IPE in and for primary care, but soon extended its scope to cover a wider spectrum for community based and later hospital-based care. Its services included provision of advice and information; responses to numerous enquiries; consultancies; reports; bulletins; workshops; and conferences. It was complemented from 1992 onwards by the *Journal of Interprofessional Care*[3] which was more wide-ranging from the outset, covering collaborative education, practice and research within and across fields of practice in the UK and, from 1997, worldwide. No less committed than CAIPE to interprofessional learning for interprofessional practice, the Journal responded also to the need to establish IPE as a disciplined activity, grounded in scholarship and worthy of a place in academe.

Debating Differences

As debates about IPE came into the open, differences in perception became more apparent within and between stakeholders: service users; pressure groups; employing agencies; professional associations; regulatory bodies; trade unions; universities and their teachers; and government departments.

Objectives

Some invoked IPE to resolve ignorance, misunderstanding and tension between practitioners from different professions, others to enhance teamwork skills, yet others to improve services, revitalise communities, remodel the workforce, or reform professional education.

Participants

Some thought that IPE should include a limited number of professions to address particular needs, opportunities or difficulties in working relationships, others that it should include the maximum practicable number.

Dosage

Some believed that a periodic IPE 'innoculation' was enough to produce a collaborative worker, others that it would only be effective if 'treatment' was sustained and pervasive.

Stage

Some held that IPE should begin on day one of pre-registration studies, continuing throughout and beyond, others that students needed time to find their respective professional identities and to put experience under their belts before being exposed to it.

Location

Some asserted that pre-registration IPE was more effective on placement, others that university and work based interprofessional learning were complementary and mutually reinforcing.

Integration

Some preferred to keep IPE on the margins of professional programmes as extra mural activities or on placement, others to weave it into the fabric of professional education programmes.

Content

Some contended that common curricula were sufficient, others holding that comparative curricula were essential for participants to explore differences as well as similarities in their values, skills and knowledge, roles and responsibilities.

Method

Some opted for one learning method, others for a repertoire on which teachers could call to address different objectives and respond to different learning needs and styles.

Planning

Some listed subjects for interprofessional teaching and learning, others preferred outcome-driven programme planning based on competencies or capabilities.

Adopting Definitions

The need for consensus about IPE became more pressing as it took on a different complexion in ever more fields of practice, prompting CAIPE to adopt the following definition and commend it to its members and more widely:

> Occasions when two or more professions learn with, from and about each other to improve collaboration and the quality of care.
>
> (CAIPE 1997)

Alive to the need to distinguish between IPE and many other occasions when health and social care professions learnt together for other reasons, it drew a distinction between IPE and multiprofessional education (MPE) defined as

> Occasions when two or more professions learn side by side for whatever reason.
>
> (CAIPE 1997)

Defined thus, IPE is a subset of MPE with permeable boundaries. It may grow within MPE in response to changes in policy or practice, or students' needs and expectations, but it may also become subsumed within MPE when its distinctive qualities are insufficiently valued and protected, especially in the face of budgetary cuts when interactive learning in small groups may seem too costly.

Enunciating Principles

Encouraged by the positive reception that these definitions had received, CAIPE took steps to reinforce them by enunciating the following principles (Box 1.1).

Box 1.1 Effective IPE

1. Works to improve the quality of care;
2. Focuses on the needs of service users and carers;
3. Involves service users and carers;
4. Encourages professions to learn with, from and about each other;
5. Respects the integrity of each profession;
6. Enhances practice within professions;
7. Increases professional satisfaction.

(CAIPE 2001)

The first of these principles is a reminder that IPE is not only grounded in practice, but also works for its improvement. The second and especially the third come through strongly in many current IPE initiatives in response to the momentum behind user-led care in UK health and social policy. The fourth reiterates the definition. The fifth and sixth are timely reminders of the need for IPE to be planned and delivered in ways that preserve and protect each profession within the wider professional family. The seventh responds to the need to cultivate mutual support to alleviate occupational stress and find fulfilment in co-working.

Classifying Learning Methods

Working with CAIPE, I distinguished between six learning methods frequently found in IPE (Box 1.2):

Box 1.2 Learning Methods in IPE

- Exchange-based learning;
  e.g. appreciative enquiry, debates, games and case studies
- Action-based learning;
  e.g. problem-based learning, collaborative enquiry and continuous quality improvement
- Practice based learning;
  e.g. training wards and co-placements
- Simulation-based learning;
  e.g. role play and experiential groups
- Observation-based learning;
  e.g. joint visits and shadowing
- Received learning;
  e.g. lectures.

(Barr 2002)

These methods are neither exhaustive nor mutually exclusive. Experienced teachers 'mix and match' them in response to different learning needs, to ring the changes and to hold the interest of their students. Received or didactic learning may be the least relevant given the stress put on interaction, but still has a place. E learning and blended learning have gained ground more recently and merit inclusion although they may be treated more appropriately as media rather than methods.

Further illumination came from the Interprofessional Education Joint Evaluation Team (JET)[4] which adopted and developed the following analysis of the characteristics of adult learning by Brookfield (1986) adding its own observations in italics:

- The adult learner is a self-directed, autonomous learner. The outcome of the learning is more likely to be positive if the learner chooses the direction, content and methods. *This poses immediate challenges for IPE. Participants may need to explore whether their perceived learning needs and desired outcomes are in harmony and whether their preferred approaches to learning coincide. Mismatches may lead to negotiation and provide excellent opportunities for collaborative learning.*
- Teachers and facilitators need to respect adult learners' needs, personalities and learning preferences. *In IPE, participants and facilitators from different professions need to accept and celebrate the diversity in the group and learn from it.*
- The experience of the learner is paramount. Life experience is both the substrata for learning and defines the particular learning needs of the individual. *Lived professional experiences, and their influence on professional attitudes and behaviour, provide bases for interprofessional exchange as participants compare perspectives and experience and sometimes challenge each other.*
- Active learning is at the heart of adult learning. *This applies especially to professional and interprofessional learning. Passive acquisition of knowledge translates poorly into practice. Active learning implies change, which may only occur if previously held attitudes and beliefs are open to challenge in a safe, supportive and co-operative learning environment.*
- Learning has to be relevant. *IPE may be instigated in response to the perceived needs of the team, the organisation, the professions or the overall service delivery system. Effective learning, however, depends upon demonstrating relevance to each participant individually.*
- Pressure to learn needs to be internalized before the participant will be motivated to learn. *Again, this is a powerful reminder that IPE, albeit designed for groups is in the final analysis, for individuals.*
- The learner needs to be ready and receptive. This may result from a degree of discomfiture, where dissonance between the desired knowledge or skill and their current state is sufficient to prompt motivation to learn and change. *Effective IPE generates such discomfort but in a supportive environment.*

(Barr *et al.* 2005: 96–97)

Responding to JET from the United States, Clarke (2006) commended interprofessional learning that was cooperative, collaborative and socially generated during exchange between the participants. It was associated with professional judgement and recognition of the social construction of knowledge within professions. Citing Kolb (1984), he saw experiential learning as a conflict-filled process out of which the development of insight, understanding and skills comes. Each profession, he said, had its cognitive or normative map derived from the process of professionalisation. IPE entailed the decentring of knowledge (Dahlgren 2006) to become aware of points of view other than one's own.

Formulating Outcomes

Given that many professional education programmes had adopted competency-based outcomes, there was a compelling argument for IPE to do likewise to facilitate its integration. Many formulations can be found in the literature, some of which were taken into account in drafting the following.

The competent practitioner will be able to do the following (Box 1.3):

Box 1.3 The Competent Practitioner

- Contribute to knowledge and development of others;
- Enable practitioners and agencies to work collaboratively to improve the effectiveness of services;
- Develop, sustain and evaluate collaborative approaches to achieve objectives;
- Contribute to the joint planning, implementation, monitoring and review of care interventions;
- Coordinate an interdisciplinary team to meet individuals' assessed needs;
- Provide assessment services on individuals' needs so that others can take action;
- Evaluate the outcome of another practitioner's assessment and care planning process.

(Barr 1998)

Some teachers questioned reliance on competency-based outcomes which they found myopic, mechanistic and reductionist, including

IPE-activists at Sheffield Hallam University who formulated instead a capability framework (Chapter 4), comprising outcomes that addressed students' ongoing learning, development and professional maturation in a working world subject to constant change and new demands.

The interprofessional team member, they said (Box 1.4):

Box 1.4 The Interprofessional Team Member

The interprofessional team member:

- is able to lead and participate in the interprofessional team and wider inter-agency work, to ensure a responsive and integrated approach to care/service management that is focused on the needs of the patient/client;
- implements an integrated assessment and plan of care/service in partnership with the patient/client, remaining responsive to the dynamics of care/service requirements;
- consistently communicates sensitively in a responsive and responsible manner, demonstrating effective interpersonal skills in the context of patient/client focused care;
- shares uniprofessional knowledge with the team in ways that contribute to and enhance service provision;
- provides a co-mentoring role to peers of own and other professions, in order to enhance service provision and personal and professional development.

(CUILU, 2004)

Checking Standards

CAIPE framed the following questions to assist in conducting internal and external checks on standards in an IPE initiative (Box 1.5):

Box 1.5 Checking Standards

- Do the aims as stated promote collaboration?
- How do the objectives contribute to collaboration?
- Do the aims and objectives contribute to improving the quality of care?
- Are aims and objectives compatible?
- How is IPE built into the programme?
- Is the programme informed by a theoretical rationale?

> **Box 1.5 (Continued)**
>
> - Is the programme evidence-based?
> - Is the programme informed by interprofessional values?
> - Does comparative learning complement common learning?
> - Are learning methods interactive?
> - Is small group learning included?
> - Will numbers from the participant professions be reasonably balanced?
> - Are all the professions represented in planning ad teaching?
> - Are service users and carers involved?
> - Will the interprofessional learning be assessed?
> - Will it count towards qualification?
> - How will the programme be evaluated?
> - Will findings be evaluated?
>
> (Barr 2003)

Challenging the Emerging Orthodoxy

These efforts to instil order into IPE were appreciated by many university teachers, but countered by commentators and researchers intent upon promoting alternative terminology and definitions (see, for example, Pirrie *et al.* 1998). Cooper and her colleagues (2004) found the packaging too tidy, commending complexity theory to provide IPE with a realistic foundation to prepare students to work in complex systems by prioritising development of skills that promoted survival and adaptation. Pressure to force IPE into 'a linear straitjacket' had to be resisted and predetermined statements of outcome set aside. Nothing could have been further removed from the challenge to the emergent IPE orthodoxy from government to which we now turn.

Embracing Government's Agenda

If 1997 marked the beginning of the road towards a unified IPE movement in the UK, it was also the year when the incoming Labour government dedicated itself to the modernisation of health and social care. From the outset, it put professional education at the heart of its strategy. Training and education (in that order) would give staff a clear understanding of how their own roles fitted with others to provide patients with integrated care. Emphasis, in the first instance, was on continuing professional development (Secretary of State for Health 1997), government judging perhaps that this would deliver change faster and encounter less resistance than attempts to reform pre-registration studies hedged about by conventions, regulations and vested interests.

But a more radical proposal followed in the NHS Plan (Secretary of State for Health 2000) in which government asserted the importance of collaboration between the NHS, higher education providers and regulatory bodies to make basic as well as post-basic education more flexible. It called for a core curriculum, comprising joint training in communication skills and in NHS principles and organisation, to promote partnerships at all levels to ensure a seamless service of patient-centred care. A new common foundation programme would give everyone working in the NHS the skills and knowledge to respond effectively to patients' individual needs, helping to give front-line staff the opportunity to think and work differently, to solve old problems in new ways and to deliver the improvements set out in the NHS Plan (Department of Health 2001). Cultivating collaboration was still on the agenda, but the salient message had become, to coin a phrase, 'educational engineering' where shared programmes would motivate and prepare students to become agents of change. Nor was that all; by 2004 government was advocating common learning to generate a more flexible workforce to further the modernisation of services, confidently asserting that attitudes were changing with 'a significant appetite for developing new roles in the services' (Department of Health 2004).

Anticipating this state of affairs, Finch (2000, cited by Barr 2002) argued that universities must understand IPE before they could embrace it. Definitions were unclear and objectives several. Was the object for students:

1. To know about the roles of other professions?
2. To be able to work with those others?
3. To be able to substitute for those others?
4. To find flexible career pathways?

With the passage of time, Finch's four objectives boil down to two:

- Learning together to improve collaborative practice.
- Learning together to build a more flexible workforce.

Implementing IPE Nationally

Implementation of each was facilitated by a different set of central organisations, the first led by the Quality Assurance Agency for Higher Education in England (QAA) and the second by Skills for Health. Insofar as both drew up frameworks and established systems for common learning, they were on the same track, but with different emphases. The QAA, and the bodies working with it, concentrated on improving collaboration between professions, based on mutual respect for identities and boundaries, seeking by common consent, to carry educational and professional interests with it. Skills for Health, whilst making passing reference to collaborative practice, concentrated on modernising the workforce in response to policy and management imperatives, less beholden than the QAA to educational and professional sensitivities.

The QAA established a series of working groups in partnership with regulatory bodies and professional associations to agree benchmarking statements to determine standards for pre-registration courses for nursing and the allied health professions (QAA 2001), social work (QAA 2000) and medicine (QAA 2002) drawn together later in a statement of common purpose (QAA 2006). The consensus achieved was remarkable and indicative of underlying moves amongst professional associations to draw closer and to find common ground, but stopping short of a formulation that might have set standards for IPE in the way that CAIPE and others had formulated. The conspicuous omission was comparative learning, the exploration of differences on which informed collaborative practice would depend to make intelligent call on the distinctive contribution of each profession. Earlier QAA work (QAA 1999) on multidisciplinary programmes was pregnant with implications for IPE, but was not brought forward. The QAA statements nevertheless proved helpful to inform the design and content of pre-registration IPE, and judgements by QAA panels reviewing IPE embedded in professional programmes. They were reinforced by the Higher Education Academy, three of whose subject centres[5] did much to promote and develop interprofessional teaching and learning, reinforced by those of the Centres for Excellence in Teaching and Learning (CETLs) which focused directly or indirectly on interprofessional learning.

'Skills for Health'[6] works with and through Strategic Health Authorities (SHAs). It has published some 60 sets of National Occupational Standards and National Workforce Competencies, based on employers' expectations for good practice in specific areas and client domains intended, amongst other purposes, to inform educational programmes and curriculum design. It has developed a Knowledge and Skills Framework within which to include them, building in ladders for career progression. It has taken steps to modernise qualifications in the healthcare sector to make them more relevant to practice and more flexible with additional points for entry and exit, secure their standards and introduce new awards such as the Foundation Degree to provide broad-based and unrestricted entry into healthcare employment. Most recently, it has put forward proposals entitled 'Equip' to standardise the monitoring of educational provision funded by SHAs on which decision, at the time of writing, had yet to be taken by government. Much of this work has been commissioned from independent consultants introducing rigour and a measure of detachment, but at the price of continuity and ongoing engagement with consultees. The imperative driving this plethora of reforms is implementation of government's workforce strategy to modernise health and social care services based upon the application of principles of human resources management where professional identities, roles and demarcations are subservient. Whilst making reference to learning for collaborative practice, it seems to be secondary to workforce reform in many Skills for Health statements.[7]

'Creating an Interprofessional Workforce' (CIPW 2007) was a three year project funded by the Department of Health to promote and develop an interprofessional culture within the health and social care workforce. Its objective was clearly to advance the modernisation agenda in association with SHAs, with whom close working relationships were established from the outset, but also with CAIPE, with whom collaboration grew closer as the project progressed. Marrying interprofessional and workforce agendas in its title, CIPW embraced both seemingly without difficulty. It succeeded, where CAIPE had failed, in engaging SHA's and NHS Trusts and other employing interests, whilst benefiting from the goodwill that CAIPE enjoyed in many universities and amongst their teachers. Given longer, with resources for follow up, CIPW might have done more to reconcile the two agendas.

Implementing IPE Locally

The road to reconciliation remained where it had always been – locally – where partnerships were established to develop 'common learning sites'. In each, responsibility for pre-registration IPE rested with one or more universities, a number of employing agencies (NHS Trusts, local authorities and from the independent sector) and the SHA. Joint management held the tension between the parties as they designed, developed, delivered and evaluated a common learning (or IPE) programme which all could own and endorse, taking into account local needs, circumstances and priorities, and implementation of national education, health and social care policies.

Albeit working from the same blueprint, development on the ground has necessarily taken many forms, depending upon topography from sparsely populated rural regions, at one extreme, to metropolitan counties and segments of London, at the other. It has taken into account historically and accidentally determined distribution of education programmes for the various health and social care professions between faculties or schools within the same and different Higher Education Institutes (HEIs) in the same and different cities. Sustainability remains problematic. Over-complex formulae for partnership falter in the face of financial and workload implications while relatively high unit costs render IPE liable to be watered down or jettisoned.

Generalisation about these developments is hazardous in the absence of a database of pre-registration IPE programmes,[8] but four 'common learning pilot sites' funded by the Department of Health have been extensively reported (Barr 2007b; Miller *et al.* 2006). Two of these sites (King's College London with Greenwich and London South Bank universities, and the Newcastle, Northumbria and Teesside universities) concentrated on developing models for interprofessional practice learning. The third (Sheffield Hallam and Sheffield universities) developed the capability framework (see above).

The fourth (Southampton and Portsmouth universities) was alone in attempting to revise curricula both to cultivate collaborative practice and to develop a more flexible workforce. Its 'New Generation Project' (NGP) remodelled the entire curriculum for pre-registration medicine, nursing, allied health professions and social work studies to comprise 'learning in common' in accordance with QAA benchmarking statements. Logistics and sheer scale precluded arranging such studies concurrently in the same classrooms or practice settings across professional groups. Instead, each group followed the same curriculam separately. Provision was, however, made for relatively short periods of intensive interactive study between the groups designed to cultivate collaboration in learning and practice. Resources have been curtailed for the long-term follow up of the NGP students. Data may therefore not be forthcoming to establish the extent to which this highly ambitious project met both objectives. Nor would it have been easy to deduce whether greater mobility in career progression or closer collaboration with other professions in practice was attributable to following the same common curriculum separately or to the time-limited intensive interprofessional learning together.

An exhaustive review of pre-registration IPE would take into account evaluations from other common learning sites. Suffice it to say that most, if not all, concentrated on preparing students for collaborative practice with few signs that workforce development was built into programme design or required outcomes. Universities have, however, responded positively to opportunities funded by SHAs to launch Foundation Degree programmes catering for a broad band of entrants to health and social care employment, and programmes for new occupational groups such as physician assistants, both of which contribute to workforce reform.

Promoting IPE Internationally

Communication and collaboration between IPE developments in the UK and other countries have progressed apace during the years under review, triggered by a seminal report from the WHO (1988) which drew on examples in developed and developing countries to inform a unifying definition and rationale for IPE.[9] Students, said the WHO, should learn together during certain periods of their education to acquire the skills necessary for solving the priority health problems of individuals and communities known to be particularly amenable to teamwork. Emphasis should be put on learning how to interact with one another, community orientation to ensure relevance to the health needs of the people and team competence.

IPE, said the WHO, should fulfil the following seven objectives (Box 1.6):

Box 1.6 Seven Objectives of IPE

1. Modify reciprocal attitudes;
2. Establish common values, knowledge and skills;
3. Build teams;

Box 1.6 (Continued)

4. Solve problems;
5. Respond to community needs;
6. Change practice;
7. Change the professions.

The first of these objectives acknowledged that ignorance, prejudice and negative stereotyping can impede effective working relations between professions, but be eased by creating opportunities to learn first hand from and about each other. The second recognised the need to establish a common foundation of values and knowledge, complemented by collaborative skills. The third treated teamwork as the primary vehicle to cultivate collaborative practice and IPE as a means to that end. The fourth accounted for the emphasis on problem-based learning (PBL) in those IPE initiatives instigated in response to the WHO lead. The fifth enlisted IPE in pursuit of a longstanding WHO objective to strengthen community based care. The sixth focused on the reform of services and the improvement of professional practice. The seventh went further, invoking IPE to change the professions from within. No one IPE initiative could realistically meet all these objectives, but many respond to one or more (Barr 2003).

Twenty years later, another WHO study group (Box 1.7) has been convened in partnership with the International Association for Interprofessional Education and Collaborative Care (InterEd):

Box 1.7 Aims of InterEd

- To review the 1988 report of the WHO Study Group on Multiprofessional Education of Health Personnel and evaluate the positive outcomes of this report as well as the areas in which little or no progress has been made;
- To assess the current state of research evidence on IPE and collaborative practice, synthesize it within an international context, and identify the gaps that must still be addressed;
- To conduct an international environmental scan to determine the current uptake of IPE and collaborative practice, discover examples that illuminate successes, barriers and enabling factors, and identify the best practices currently known in this area;

- To develop a conceptual framework that would identify the key issues that must be considered and addressed by WHO and its partners when formulating a global operational plan for IPE and collaborative practice;
- To identify, evaluate and synthesize evidence on the potential facilitators, incentives and levers for action that could be recommended as part of a global strategy for IPE and collaborative practice.

(Yan *et al.* 2007)

It is clear from deliberations, so far, that impact from this second IPE report within WHO will depend upon addressing its two overriding concerns: first, application of lessons learned from IPE in developed countries to developing countries and, second, the relevance of IPE to the WHO's strategy to tackle the global crisis in the number, distribution and deployment of skilled personnel in the healthcare workforce (WHO 2006). Much the same pressure may then be building up internationally as nationally to enlist IPE as an agent of workforce reform.

There is, however, nothing in the international literature of IPE (Barr 2005) to suggest that workforce objectives have been included. Findings from systematic reviews must be treated with extreme caution, based on highly selected examples of IPE initiatives subjected to robust evaluation. The Interprofessional JET scanned over 10,000 reports of IPE evaluations from which it selected 107 to include in its first analysis (Barr *et al.* 2005) and 21 in its second adopting a higher threshold (Hammick *et al.* 2007). It classified outcomes as follows based on a modification of the scale devised by Kirkpatrick (1967) for vocational training (Table 1.1):

Table 1.1 The JET Classification of IPE Outcomes

Level 1 – Reaction	Learners' views on the learning experience and its interprofessional nature.
Level 2a – Modification of attitudes/perceptions	Changes in reciprocal attitudes or perceptions between participant groups. Changes in perception or attitude towards the value and/or use of team approaches to caring for a specific client group.
Level 2b – Acquisition of knowledge/skills	Including knowledge and skills linked to interprofessional collaboration.

Table 1.1 Continued

Level 3 – Behavioural change	Identifies individuals' transfer of interprofessional learning to their practice setting and their changed professional practice.
Level 4a – Change in organisational practice	Wider changes in the organisation and delivery of care.
Level 4b – Benefits to patients/clients	Improvements in health or wellbeing of patients/clients.

Based on its analysis, JET distinguished between three overlapping types of IPE by primary focus:

1. Preparing the individuals for collaborative practice;
2. Developing teamwork;
3. Improving services.

The first of these applied most strongly to pre-registration IPE and the third to work based IPE between experienced practitioners. The second was under-represented at both stages, despite much lip service paid to teambuilding in the interprofessional literature.

JET's working definition for IPE focused on learning for collaborative practice. It made no reference to developing a more flexible workforce. Examples of learning together with that focus might have been missed. Account must also be taken of the time lag between initiatives being conducted and evaluated, and a systematic review reporting. It may well be prudent therefore to allow for the possibility that learning together for health and social care professions has developed more recently. Furthermore, it might characterise such learning in developing countries underrepresented in the IPE literature and absent from systematic reviews.

Conclusion

Despite sustained endeavours to instil coherence, IPE remains a 'broad church'. That may be its strength, provided that systems for planning, delivery and evaluation are robust enough to reconcile different objectives operationally. At issue is whether IPE and common learning are one and the same, or whether the former is qualitatively different to be embedded within the latter, following the Southampton/Portsmouth model.

For common learning to pave the way for substitution and career progression, it needs either to be taught to the same level across the constituent professions or topped up as necessary. Either way, it needs to be applied to different roles in different work settings.

For interprofessional learning to cultivate collaborative practice, it needs not only common but also comparative curricula, complemented by interactive, exchange-based learning methods. Logistics and costs may dictate that it remains a relatively small proportion of the overall study time compared to the common learning within which it is embedded. This puts a premium on its potency, but its impact may depend also upon the extent to which its values and insights come to characterise both the common and the profession-specific learning.

Much remains to be done to reconcile these two agendas, once their different objectives and implications for content and learning methods are better understood and stakeholders locally, nationally and internationally engage.

Notes

1. The term 'service user' did not gain currency for another 20 years.
2. www.caipe.org.uk.
3. www.informahealthcare.com.
4. All of whom were active members of CAIPE.
5. Health Sciences and Practice, Medicine, Dentistry and Veterinary Medicine, and Social Work and Social Policy.
6. With 'Skills for Care' as agents of central government working with Strategic Health Authorities, human resources management in NHS trusts and local authorities.
7. See www.skillsforhealth.org.uk.
8. Numerous national reviews of IPE up to 1997 (summarised in Barr 2007b), all reported before these programmes were established.
9. The WHO preferred the term MPE at that time, but accorded the same meaning as the term IPE, which it later adopted.

References

Barr, H. (1998). Competent to collaborate: Towards a competency-based model for interprofessional education. *Journal of Interprofessional Care* 12 (2), 181–188.

Barr, H. (2002). *Interprofessional Education: Today, Yesterday and Tomorrow*. London: LTSN Health Sciences and Practice.

Barr, H. (2003). Ensuring quality in interprofessional education. *CAIPE Bulletin* 22, 2–3.

Barr, H. (2005) Learning together. In G. Meads and J. Ashcroft *et al.* (eds) *The Case for Interprofessional Education in Health and Social Care.* Oxford: Blackwell.

Barr, H. (2007a). *Interprofessional Education in the United Kingdom: 1966 to 1997.* London: Higher Education Academy, Health Sciences & Practice, Occasional Paper 9.

Barr, H. (ed.) (2007b). *Piloting Interprofessional Education: Four English Case Studies.* London: Higher Education Academy Health Sciences and Practice Subject Centre.

Barr, H. (2008). *Conservative and Transformative Agenda for Interprofessional Education: Squaring the Circle.* Keynote address: All Together Better Health Four, Stockholm, 3 June.

Barr, H., I. Koppel, S. Reeves, M. Hammick, and D. Freeth. (2005). *Effective Interprofessional Education: Argument, Assumption and Evidence.* Oxford: Blackwell.

Brookfield, S. (1986). *Understanding and Facilitating Adult Learning: A Comprehensive Analysis of Principles and Effective Practice.* Milton Keynes: Open University Press.

CAIPE. (1997). Interprofessional education – A definition. *CAIPE Bulletin* 13, 19.

CAIPE. (2001). *Principles of Interprofessional Education.* London: CAIPE.

CIPW. (2007). *Creating an Interprofessional Workforce: An Education and Training Framework for Health and Social Care in England.* London: Department of Health with CAIPE.

Clarke, P. (2006). What would a theory of interprofessional education look like? Some suggestions for developing a theoretical framework for teamwork training. *Journal of Interprofessional Care* 20 (6), 577–590.

Cooper, H., S. Braye, and R. Geyer. (2004). Complexity and interprofessional education. *Learning for Health and Social Care* 3 (4), 45–52.

CUILU. (2004). *Interprofessional Capability Framework.* Sheffield: Combined Universities Interprofessional Learning Unit.

Dahlgren, L. (2006). *Developing Practice Through Experiencing Variety: A Potential Function of Interprofessional Learning for Improving Competence.* Paper presented to the All Together Better Health III conference, London, April.

Department of Health. (2001). *A Health Service for All the Talents: Developing the NHS Workforce.* London: Department of Health.

Department of Health. (2004). *The NHS Knowledge and Skills Framework (NHS KSF) and the Development Review Process.* London: Department of Health.

Finch, J. (2000). Interprofessional education and teamworking; A view from the educational provider. *British Medical Journal* 312, 1138–1140.

Hallett, C. and E. Birchall. (1992). *Co-Ordination and Child Protection: A Review of the Literature.* Edinburgh: HMSO.

Hammick, M., D. Freeth, S. Reeves, I. Koppel, and H. Barr. (2007). *A Best Evidence Systematic Review of Interprofessional Education.* Dundee: Best Evidence Medical Education.

Kirkpatrick, D. (1967). Evaluation of training. In R. Craig and L. Bittel (eds) *Training and Development Handbook.* New York: McGraw-Hill, pp. 87–112.

Kolb, D. (1984). *Experiential Learning.* Englewood Cliffs, NJ: Prentice-Hall.

Miller, C., C. Woolf, and N. Mackintosh. (2006). *Evaluation of Common Learning Pilots and Allied Health Professions First Wave Sites* (Final report). Brighton: University of Brighton for the Department of Health.

Pirrie, A., V. Wilson, R. Harden, and J. Elsegood. (1998). Promoting cohesive practice in health care. *AMEE Guide & Medical Teacher* 20 (5), 409–416.

QAA. (1999). *Benchmarking Academic Standards: The Advisory Group on Multidisciplinary and Modular Programmes: Final Report.* Bristol: Quality Assurance Agency for Higher Education.

QAA. (2000). *Social Policy and Administration and Social Work: Subject Benchmarking Statements.* Bristol: Quality Assurance Agency for Higher Education.

QAA. (2001). *Benchmarking Academic and Practitioner Standards in Health Care Subjects.* Bristol: Quality Assurance Agency for Higher Education.

QAA. (2002). *Medicine: Subject Benchmarking Statements.* Bristol: Quality Assurance Agency for Higher Education.

QAA. (2006). *Statement of Common Purpose for Subject Benchmarks Statements for Health and Social Care Professions.* Bristol: Quality Assurance Agency for Higher Education.

Secretary of State for Health. (1997). *The New NHS; Modern; Dependable.* London: Department of Health.

Secretary of State for Health. (2000). *The NHS Plan.* London: The Stationery Office.

WHO. (1988). *Learning Together to Work Together for Health.* Geneva: World Health Organization.

WHO. (2006). *Working Together for Health: The World Health Report.* Geneva: World Health Organization.

Yan, J., J. Gilbert, and S. Hoffman. (2007). World Health Organization study group on interprofessional education and collaborative practice. *Journal of Interprofessional Care* 21 (6), 587.

2

Interprofessional Education: Unpacking the Early Challenges

Patricia Bluteau and Ann Jackson

Introduction

In the previous chapter, Barr offers a reminder within the UK that early initiatives first emerged in the sixties. It is incredible to consider that we are approaching 50 years of drive to implement interprofessional education (IPE) across health and social care groups. So after all this time why does it feel that IPE is still being perceived as a new and troublesome concept?

Mhaolrunaigh argues that IPE '... as a concept and new paradigm has increasingly developed partisanship since the early seventies' (Mhaolrunaigh 2001: 1) and certainly it would appear that change has been slow and that the drive for interprofessional integration has lacked sufficient positive drivers. The early practice based initiatives that were often prey to the rocky complexities of working within health and social care currently still resonate.

This chapter will build on Barr's opening chapter, by exploring further the climate in which IPE developed in the late twentieth and early twenty-first centuries. It will concentrate on the challenges that were evident in the early days of IPE, when development was patchy and fragmented. It will focus on the climate in higher education institutes (HEIs) and the impact of the early introduction of IPE, which engineered the development of collaborative approaches across and between organisations. Chapter 3 will bring the reader up to date by providing a current picture of IPE in HEIs.

Background

The emphasis on modernisation has dominated the National Health Service (NHS) especially towards the end of the twentieth and into the twenty-first centuries. This agenda has charged health and social care professionals with delivering an efficient, effective and quality service. This has had to occur within a finite allocation of resources which has not only served to make the process more difficult but also resulted in professional groups raising concerns in relation to maintaining and improving their own status. For instance, the move from schools of nursing to higher education institutions possibly increased the gap between the needs of the NHS, in terms of skills, teams and roles, in its pursuit to increase both the academic and professional status of nursing.

The government's emphasis on delivering care starting with the patient's needs demanded a climate of good teamworking and an understanding of patient-centred care (DH 2002). Not with what, some might say, was a misdirected emphasis on the pursuit of uniprofessional academic reward.

Catastrophes within the public eye only served to increase the call for educating professionals together, in the hope of removing the stereotypes and attitudes held by professionals, but this reduced further the autonomy and independence of many professions, which, in turn, hindered effective teamwork (Pietroni 1994; Laming Report 2003; Shipman Inquiry 2005).

In 1984 the World Health Organisation (WHO) identified that professional education should work towards enhancing working relationships (WHO 1984). Yet it took another decade for developments in policy to clarify how working together could improve the experience of the patient.

> Integrated care for patients will rely on models of training and education that give staff a clear understanding of how their own roles fit with those of others within both the health and social care professions. The government will work with the professions to reach a shared understanding of the principles that should underpin effective continuing professional development and the respective roles of the state, the professionals and individual practitioners in supporting this activity.
>
> (Department of Health 1997: Paragraph 6.10)

The need for integrated teams to deliver this care was highlighted, as was the need for education and training to ensure the teams had the appropriate skills and knowledge. Historically, each profession had its own training and funding but efforts were made to explore ways of drawing professionals together, for educational and resource reasons.

With the development of health improvement plans (DH 1999) the need for integration became one step closer. It became obvious that no one professional group had all the necessary skills and knowledge to deliver care; therefore multiprofessional teams were a necessity. Collaboration became a necessity. The uniprofessional model of training did not fit with a health policy which put the patient experience at the centre of care, where communication and liaison were key elements of delivering quality care (Leathard 2003).

The later development of national service frameworks (NSFs) (DH 2000) brought professional and governmental bodies together. The collaboration of a range of experts, drawn from across professional boundaries, acted as another step towards forging the need to understand and respect each other's professional roles in delivering quality care. Development of each of the NSFs involved identification of any training or educational needs which lent itself to shared learning. Implicit within the frameworks was also the notion of treatment by multiprofessional specialist teams.

As the modernisation programme kicked in, it became apparent that many of the proposed changes depended on existing staff extending, or in some cases developing new roles, in order to develop a flexible workforce. In particular, developing new skills, taking on new roles and working outside traditional boundaries needed to be encouraged and rewarded rather than regarded as inappropriate. This required changes in education and training, in regulation and in employment practices, as well as a willingness to embrace change among all bodies including staff representatives (DH 2002).

Traditional demarcation lines between professional groups and between professional and non-professional groups (e.g. between doctors and nurses or between nurses and health care assistants) were not conducive to delivering high-quality, patient-centred care.

Barr comments, in Chapter 1, that even today the notion of a flexible workforce is '*ill understood and ill addressed*'. A '*flexible workforce*' was seen by many professionals as a potential for deskilling – for example, physician assistants, surgical assistants, emergency care practitioners and so on, and may have served to create some hostility or at least caution to the implementation of IPE.

McGrath (1991) offered an alternative perspective to this, one that concentrated on a confident, capable professional, able to embrace their colleagues' contributions on an equal footing so patient care would benefit:

> Interprofessional working is not about fudging the boundaries between the professions and trying to create a generic care worker. It is instead about developing professionals who are confident in their own core skills and expertise, who are fully aware and confident in the skills and expertise of fellow health and care professionals, and who conduct their own practice in a non-hierarchical and collegiate way with other members of the working team, so as to continuously improve the health of their communities and to meet the real care needs of individual patients and clients.
>
> (McGrath 1991)

We would argue that the wariness of IPE persists to this day but we clearly see IPE as a vehicle which allows professions to celebrate the unique aspects of their professional identity whilst embracing and acknowledging the boundaries and overlap between professions. Meads and Ashcroft (2005) would support this by emphasising that this method of learning enhances the collaborative culture.

Setting the scene in Higher Education

For those involved in IPE today, the issues and challenges to the development, implementation and evaluation are thorny and at times intractable. In the early nineties authors reported the advantages and disadvantages of IPE initiatives in higher education (HE) (Tope 1994; Casto 1994; Knapp and associates 1998). The overwhelming message of concern from these authors appeared to relate to a lack of resources and commitment, to be able to implement IPE effectively, both within practice and education settings.

Knapp succinctly states,

> Interprofessional programmes within universities...operate in an environment that is in varying degrees indifferent or even hostile, to the enterprise.
>
> (Knapp *et al.* 1998: 19)

> Collaborative efforts in IPE 'immediately stretch(es) individuals from both inside and outside the university walls beyond their comfort zone'.
>
> (Knapp *et al.* 1998: 198)

Historically, perhaps, it was this that was responsible for creating a divide between those lecturers who became champions of IPE and those who did not. Champions were able to embrace the notion that IPE aimed to improve client care and were able to bridge the theory/practice divide unlike those who believed that the introduction of IPE was merely change for change sake (Mhaolrunaigh 2001).

It was fortunate in many ways that champions emerged so quickly, given the Department of Health's (1994) challenge to education providers to exploit opportunities for shared learning and to place the emphasis on student-focused and practice-led initiatives.

One of the main problems regarding the education of health and social care professionals was that learning predominantly ran in parallel rather than in tandem (McCroskey and Einbinder 1998). Traditional approaches to educating health and social care professionals did not promote collaborative practice (Leathard 1994), but why should they, as they had been developed to encourage an immersion into one chosen profession. This led to immense tension, as barriers were erected to preserve uniprofessional space.

A proposed model of undergraduate IPE was quickly condemned in HEIs due to logistics, and the cry from lecturers that students could not learn from and about each other when they did not learn together either in university or in practice (Barr 1994). Barr further counselled that the impact of large groups had not been taken into account, in terms of their needs and levels of satisfaction, and that in reality the high priority of HEIs was the need to reduce cost and repetition of work.

Whilst these challenges were associated with early developments in IPE, they are still current and relevant today with organisational and administrative tensions (Gilbert 2005), communication and service demand pressures (Jackson and Bluteau 2007), professional cultural beliefs and logistics (Barker *et al.* 2005). In many ways the very nature of the struggle in the early drive to implement IPE has strengthened the early challenges, and they remain in some cases, intractable and deep seated.

However, with the political and professional imperative gaining momentum, HEIs were required to consider how they would incorporate IPE into the curriculum. As this affected all institutions it forced multiple HEIs to collaborate and find ways of delivering IPE to both undergraduate and postgraduate health and social care learners. There are many complex and interrelated issues in cross institutional collaboration; most commonly, these relate to the impact of differing priorities and motivation at individual, team and institutional level. The colliding priorities of different institutions only served to enhance the challenges.

Development of the Role of the Lecturer

Lecturers' views regarding the teaching of IPE have been categorised in two separate ways, first that lecturers believed that IPE was *'potentially the correct thing to do'* and second that it was *'politically the correct thing to do'* (Mhaolrunaigh 2001: 236). Lecturers needed convincing that their aim in facilitating IPE was to *'breakdown boundaries, dissolve tribalism and resolve conflict'* (Mhaolrunaigh 2001: 239), but their poor understanding of the principles of IPE clearly highlighted the difficulties of attempting to try to embed a new overarching concept into an existing uniprofessional structure. Little thought had been given to the impact on *'human and physical resources or sufficient advance planning'*. Not surprisingly, lecturers were left with different degrees of disillusionment and frustration. For IPE to work 'first and foremost', teachers needed to believe in it, understand it and demonstrate solidarity 'as ambassadors' (Mhaolrunaigh 2001: 237).

As early as 1986, Jones recommended the importance of teachers being exposed to the same collaborative learning style as their students, in order that they might learn from, and through, their experience. This was supported by Mhaolrunaigh (2001) who concurred that not only should teachers be exposed to this style of teaching, but also that they learn the overarching concepts of IPE and learn *'how to deal with groups of mixed composition'* (Mhaolrunaigh 2001: 236).

However, those lecturers leading IPE found themselves in a tricky position as they were dependent on colleagues not involved in the development of the IPE component of the course, to commit to, and facilitate, IPE activities. IPE champions were also faced with colleagues who were concerned about the perceived conflict between maintaining professional autonomy and the dilution of boundaries between the professional groups, creating tensions and opposition in the delivery and facilitation of IPE (Julia and Thompson 1994; Barker *et al.* 2005; Howkins and Bray 2008).

Challenging Professional Cultures

The proliferation of 'separatist' or 'silo' models within undergraduate curricula in the early days of IPE was endemic within professional education. Historically, there has always been a division, between the health and social care sectors (Hugman 1995). Health and social care sectors emerge from different backgrounds and philosophies and as such view themselves as 'different' to each other. Within IPE, the intention was to celebrate, not discard, these differences.

The consequences of these uniprofessional models led to teamwork being expounded in terms of the uniprofessional team, rather than the potential for the overlapping of boundaries with other professional groups, which was the premise of interprofessional model (Clark 1993).

It might seem that the IPE stance endorsed by Barr (1994) of advocating collaborative working made overwhelming sense in the light of holistic client care, yet the deeply entrenched silo model remained much respected in the early nineties, and still has some strong advocates today (Barker *et al.* 2005), who remain keen to maintain their status resulting in a refusal to accept any positive aspects of IPE.

Even today the underlying culture of professional groups is such that primary professional groups, of which medicine is one, enjoy and are rewarded by the public with high status, esteem and financial rewards. Most other professions within the NHS – Nursing, Occupational Therapy, Physiotherapy and other allied health and social care professionals – have until recently been regarded as secondary professions; today they are deemed to have achieved professional status.

Professions, by their very being, create their own professional codes and regulatory bodies which act to police and maintain the integrity and structure of their professional set as well as maintaining the hierarchy. Through maintaining control over their own knowledge base and qualifications they are able to maintain occupational status. The evidence of this hierarchical structure within health and social care groups immediately causes constraints in terms of collaborative endeavours. Furthermore, silo models do not lend themselves towards a collaborative model of education; indeed the very nature of professional groups is to maintain their higher status, by ensuring that the public believes that their work is more vital to society than that of other professional groups. Within this context IPE could be viewed (and probably is by some) as a dumbing down or at worse the loss of some important uniprofessional knowledge (in order to make room for generic knowledge). Such beliefs, held by many professionals, make the silo or uniprofessional model hard to give up. The consequence of changing from a silo model to a collaborative one is therefore difficult and requires flexibility and motivation.

Mhaolrunaigh (2001: 25) suggests that IPE requires students to undertake two transitions to work collaboratively. First, they need to reflect upon their own profession recognising their own professional background, and second, to 'reflect and recognise their own profession in relation to new others within the group'. We would argue that this is equally applicable to facilitators if they wish to leave the silo model behind.

The problems of terminology

Whilst professional status has caused problems, communication between different groups of health care professionals has been severely hindered by the diversity of language used within professional groupings (Pietroni 1992). Work undertaken by Pietroni (1992) concluded that links between language, thought, culture and ideology needed to be addressed within health professional groups, if uniprofessional boundaries were to be crossed.

Each professional group developed value systems and specialist language known and owned by its members, such that 'ownership of status and role identification was of utmost importance' in ensuring the separatist professional model was maintained (Mhaolrunaigh 2001). Possessing profession-specific jargon fosters feelings of superiority and safety within individual groups, but can be damaging for the patient who may receive the same information from different professional groups, each using a different language. Mhaolrunaigh (2001) drawing on the work of Kuhn (1970) suggested that if knowledge is 'intrinsically the common property of a group or else nothing at all' (Kuhn 1970: 210) then perhaps all that is needed is a common language for health and social care professional groups. This could be attained through interprofessional working which, in turn, might help patients become empowered in their care.

Working Towards Collaboration

Collaboration at all levels is difficult. It involves a willingness to change and requires participating institutions to make explicit the value base from which they are engaging. Where such collaboration occurs it is associated with positive outcomes (Barr 2007). Further evidence supports this and demonstrates that when multiple HEIs collaborate, knowledge and understanding of education practices, in any given field, occurs (Howkins and Bray 2008).

Howkins and Bray (2008) did however identify that in order to maximise collaborative learning, expert facilitation is essential. This directly opposes the assumptions that professionals can readily facilitate effective IPE on the basis of their expertise as a practitioner or lecturer. Most professionals incorporate teaching and mentoring whilst carrying high workloads; to add IPE to this heavy burden without ensuring that they possess the necessary level of facilitation skills is dooming them to failure. To make this even more difficult there is often little or no funding for IPE in practice.

Facilitation is not the only challenge to implementing IPE, further challenges lie in the teaching and learning strategies.

In the early nineties as efforts to collaborate took shape, a new vocabulary of 'shared learning', 'common learning' and 'collaborative learning' began to emerge. Internationally, 'shared learning' within an educational context was used as an umbrella term (Tope 1994; Knapp and associates 1998) to describe the whole range of teaching and learning activities associated with students learning together, but did little to provide a consensus over exactly what IPE was. This was probably because models of collaboration and shared learning covered such a wide range of possibilities, combining varying amounts of theory and practice, course design, learning outcomes, assessment and final awards. Professional bodies (ENB/CCETSW 1995) began to explore the range of possibilities in terms of shared learning, which would act as a precursor to later IPE initiatives.

One of the major stumbling blocks associated with shared learning was, and in some cases still is, that it is seen as a poisoned chalice, one that removes an individual's professional autonomy and encourages professionals in a climate of limited resources to share lectures that don't quite meet any profession-specific need. For example, critics of the common foundation programme in nursing criticised the use of shared learning across the branches of nursing as the largest branch tended to dominate the focus of the lectures, thus marginalising and possibly devaluing the smaller branches.

In many instances shared learning was viewed as simply putting different professional groups together in a single room, to learn side by side without sharing professional philosophies, knowledge and cultures. Shaw (1994) argued that it could only be properly termed 'shared learning' if it included interactive learning that drew on the past experiences and background knowledge of the participants. Clark (1993) further showed that participants who had undertaken shared learning should be able to break down obstructive stereotypes through the process of working together and being able to identify their shared skills and values. Sharing this understanding could develop greater understanding of each other's roles and lead to the development of productive working relationships provided that the shared learning initiatives were carefully thought out and planned. Clarification of 'shared learning' was desperately needed. In 1993 Clark provided this with a shared learning hierarchy (Box 2.1).

Box 2.1 Shared Learning Hierarchy

- Unidisciplinary – where one professional group learns from each other (within their own profession) to understand a specific body of knowledge.
- Multidisciplinary – where several professions are exposed to the same material, in parallel rather than at the same time, or place.
- Interdisciplinary or interprofessional – often used interchangeably but indicating learning where students from different professional backgrounds communicate together to share their thoughts regarding their work.

(Clark 1993)

Clark's description of multidisciplinary and IPE was extended by Leathard (1994). She suggested that IPE should be viewed as a shared context between health and social care professions, whilst multidisciplinary education should refer to a much wider range of academic disciplines outside of the realms of health and social care.

In 1997 the Centre for the Advancement of Interprofessional Education (CAIPE) offered a definition of IPE, which provided clarity and a way forward for health and social care professionals and educationalists (Chapter 1) and which is now internationally accepted.

Concluding thoughts

Since those early days it is recognised now, in terms of 'teaching' within IPE, that lecturers need to take on a facilitation role in which they foster and encourage collaborative working between student professionals rather than using didactic teaching methods (Howkins and Bray 2008). Bruffee (1999) drawing on the work of Kuhn (1970) examines the issues surrounding the development of collaborative working between students and facilitators:

Collaborative learning is a reacculturative process that helps students become members of knowledge communities whose common property is different from the common property of the knowledge communities they already belong to.

(Bruffee 1993: 3)

Facilitators need to be able to enable an interprofessional group to develop a common language. Collaborative learning will occur as the intellectual judgement switches from the lecturer being in control and holding power within the group to a climate in which the social, emotional and intellectual relationships between the group members take precedence. Lecturers can have an impact on this process not in terms of teaching 'knowledge' but by creating conditions that will allow students to cross the boundaries from passivity to empowerment within the group (Dewey 1938). By facilitating the group to develop self-direction and independence, students are able to begin learning collaboratively together. There is some evidence that this is a problem at pre-qualifying level because students at this level can place high demands on teacher time and 'knowledge' expecting to be taught, rather than creating learning climates for themselves with minimal lecturer intervention (Wall 1994). In part this may be due to students coming straight from school environments where high levels of support are given, which may result in a concrete approach to learning which requires further development and extension within a higher education context. Such a style of learning may cause problems in terms of collaborative learning expectations, especially in the early years of pre-qualifying courses.

Bruffee (1993) supports the need for facilitation by directly opposing traditional notions of the authority of knowledge, lectures and institutions. He believes that learning occurs among people, and not between people. The work on collaborative learning of Bruffee (1993) is useful in terms of IPE, as it implies that it is possible for diverse groups of health and social care professional communities to work together collaboratively. In addition, learning becomes a new type of interaction, in which new communities form and new community knowledge is developed. Students within new communities are able to develop interdependence to function within their new community and so develop an understanding of each other within this new environment.

Conclusion

The changing emphasis of government legislation regarding health and social care policy clearly impacted on the development of IPE. This chapter has explored the difficulties and challenges faced by IPE in the nineties, concentrating on the emerging pedagogy which is helping to shape the development of IPE today. Although some of these challenges can still be seen today, the developing transparency evolving within IPE communities offers valuable support to individuals looking to develop IPE activities.

References

Barker, K.K., K. Bosco, and I.F. Oandasan. (2005). Factors in implementing inter-professional education and collaborative practice initiatives: Findings from key informant interviews. *Journal of Interprofessional Care* (May) 19 (Suppl. 1), 166–176.

Barr, H. (1994). *Perspectives on Shared Learning*. London: CAIPE.

Barr, H. (ed.) (2007). *Piloting Interprofessional Education: Four English Case Studies*. London: Higher Education Academy Health Sciences and Practice Subject Centre.

Bruffee, K.A. (1999). *Collaborative Learning: Higher Education, Interdependence, and the Authority of Knowledge*, 2nd edn. London; Baltimore, MD: Johns Hopkins University Press.

CAIPE. (1997). Interprofessional education – A definition. *CAIPE Bulletin* 13, 19.

Casto, M. (1994). Interprofessional work in the USA – education and practice, in Clark, P.G. (1993), *Journal of Interprofessional Care* 7 (3), 219–220.

Department of Health. (1994). *Nursing Midwifery and Health Visiting Education: A Statement of Strategic Intent*. Lancashire: DOH.

Department of Health. (1997). *The New NHS: Modern Dependable*. London: Department of Health, The Stationery Office.

Department of Health. (1999). The Health Act. HImP. *A First Class Service*. London: Department of Health, The Stationery Office.

Department of Health. (2000). *The NHS Plan*. London: Department of Health, The Stationery Office.

Department of Health. (2002). *Liberating the Talents: Helping Primary Care Trusts and Nurses to Deliver the NHS Plan*. London: Department of Health, The Stationery Office.

Dewey, J. (1938). *Experience and Education*. New York: The Macmillan company.

ENB/CCETSW (1995). *Shared Learning: A Good Practice Guide*.

Gilbert, J.H.V. (2005). Interprofessional learning and higher education structural barriers. *Journal of Interprofessional Care* 19 (Suppl. 1), 87–106.

Howkins, E. and J. Bray. (2008). *Preparing for Interprofessional Teaching: Theory and Practice*. Oxford: Radcliffe.

Hugman, R. (1995). Contested territories and community services: Interprofessional boundaries in health and social care. In Soothill, K., Mackay, L. and Webb, C. (eds), *Interprofessional Relations in Health Care*. London: Edward Arnold, pp. 31–45.

Jackson, J.A. and P.A.S. Bluteau. (2007). At first it's like shifting sands: Setting up interprofessional learning within a secondary care setting. *Journal of Interprofessional Care* 21 (3) June, 351–353.

Jones, R. (1986). Working together – learning together, *Journal of the Royal College of General Practitioners* 33, 1–26.

Julia, M.C. and A. Thompson. (1994). Group process and interprofessional teamwork. In Castro, R.M., Julia, M.C., Platt, L.J., Harbaugh, G.L., Waugaman, W.R., Thompson, A., Jost, T.S., Bope, E.T., Williams, T. and Lee, D.B. (eds), *Interprofessional Care and Collaborative Practice*. Pacific Grove: Brooks/Cole.

Knapp, M. and Associates. (1998). *Paths to Partnership: University and Community as Learners in Interprofessional Education*. Maryland, USA: Rowman & Littlefield Publishers Inc.

Kuhn, T. (1970). *The Structure of Scientific Revolutions*, 2nd edn. Chicago: The University of Chicago Press.

Laming Report (2003). http://www.victoria-climbie-inquiry.org.uk/finreport/finreport.htm, accessed 30 January 2009.

Leathard, A. (ed.) (1994). *Going Inter-professional: Working Together for Health and Welfare*. London: Routledge.

Leathard, A. (2003). Chapter 2: Policy Overview. In Leathard, A. (ed.), *Interprofessional Collaboration: From Policy to Practice in Health and Social Care*. East Sussex: Brunner Routledge.

McCroskey, M.J. and Einbinder, S.D. (eds) (1998). *Universities and Communities Remaking Professional and Interprofessional Education for the Next Century*. Westport: Praeger.

McGrath, M. (1991). *Multi-disciplinary Teamwork: Community Mental Handicap Teams*. Brookfield: Gower Publishing Company.

Meads, G. and J. Ashcroft. (2005). In Meads, G. and Ashcroft, J. (eds), *The Case for Interprofessional Collaboration in Health and Social Care*. Oxford: Blackwell Publishing Ltd.

Mhaolrunaigh, S.N. (2001). An evaluation of interprofessional education for health and social care professionals: The teachers' views. PhD Thesis, University of Warwick.

Pietroni, P.C. (1992). Towards reflective practice – the languages of health and social care. *Journal of Interprofessional Care* 6 (1), 7–16.

Pietroni, P. (1994). Interprofessional teamwork: Its history and development in hospitals, general practice and community care (UK). In Leathard, A. (ed.), *Going Interprofessional: Working Together for Health and Welfare*. London: Routledge.

Shaw, I. (1994). *Evaluating Interprofessional Training*. Avebury: Aldershot.

The Shipman Inquiry (2005). http://www.the-shipman-inquiry.org.uk/home.asp, accessed 30 January 2009.

Tope, R. (1994). *Integrated Interdisciplinary Learning Between Health and Social Care Professions: A Feasibility Study*. PhD Thesis, University of Wales.

Wall, J.M. (1994). *Mentoring Relationships in Initial Nurse Education*. MA Thesis, University of Warwick.

WHO (1984). *Education and Training of Nursing Nurse Teachers and Managers with Special Regards to Primary Health Care*. Report of a WHO committee technical report series 780 Geneva.

3

Interprofessional Education in Higher Education Institutions: Models, Pedagogies and Realities

Helen Langton

Introduction

The evolving use of interprofessional learning (IPL) in the higher education setting has become more prevalent over the last 8–10 years. This has led to a variety of typologies or models evolving over this time as academics seek new and innovative ways to embed IPL in a meaningful and sustainable way. In addition, these models have taken differing approaches to the philosophies and beliefs regarding learning, teaching and assessment that have underpinned them.

This chapter will open with an examination of the definitions of IPL that have been either developed or adopted in higher education institutions (HEIs). Alongside this will be a discussion regarding the placing of IPL related to stages of curriculum and professional development. The chapter will then explore five current models in use, using case studies from a number of HEIs. The approaches to learning, teaching and assessment will also be outlined. For each model there are benefits and challenges relating to management of IPL and these will be identified and a discussion offered and, where possible, solutions identified.

Definitions and Aims of Interprofessional Learning

The growing body of literature related to IPL has one striking factor in common regardless of what is being shared or profiled. The definition of IPL continues to dominate each paper as authors debate words such as multiprofessional, interprofessional, shared learning and common learning. Definitions range from the WHO (1987) that state that multiprofessional education is

> the process by which a group of students (or workers) from the health related occupations with different educational backgrounds learn together during certain periods of their education with interaction as an important goal, to collaborate in providing promotive, preventative, rehabilitative and other health related services.
>
> (WHO 1987: 6)

It is commonly cited as a starting point but rarely the point of completion of the debate. Many also cite the search terms used by the Zwarenstein *et al.* (2000) systematic review. Many see the terms as synonymous, but for others they represent clear distinctions and lead to different pedagogical models being used to develop different types of learning. The Department of Health (DH) added confusion to the debate as, in policy documents, they refer constantly to common learning (2001), to describe the provision of opportunities for students of different professions to learn together.

Some authors, for example Miller, Freeman and Ross (2001), identify common learning as the sharing of common content or the teaching of core skills and this would resonate with Barr's definition of multiprofessional learning (CAIPE 1997).

More frequently, the literature resonates with the CAIPE definition of IPL as being

> Learning with, from and about each other
>
> (CAIPE 1997),

although not always going on to identify that this is in order to facilitate collaboration and improve the quality of care (Barr 2002).

Whilst the debate continues to engage academics and practitioners alike, more recent literature does begin to demonstrate a commonality of use of terms. So, for example, common or shared learning begins to resonate with learning whereby the content is shared but the thrust or focus is not on learning with, from and about each other. However, it serves to ensure that common learning outcomes, often related to key content areas such as research and evidence-based practice, ethics or communication, are identified across professional groups. In addition, this common content across a range of professional groups may or may not be taught together, partly due to whether this produces economies of scale, the environmental resources available (if this is to large groups) and other constraining factors such as timetabling.

In addition, there also appears to be consensus in relation to the definition of interprofessional as learning which involves 'with, from and about each other'; and consensus that the aim of undertaking this is for a focus which may include the development of one or more of the following:

- skills for collaborative working;
- teamwork;
- enhancement of patient care;
- interprofessional attitudes;
- understanding of roles.

Finally, there is also clarity that curriculum continues to include elements of uniprofessional learning and, when explored in detail it is clear that in many of the models being explored in this chapter, uniprofessional learning still carries the majority of weight within the curriculum.

It is clear then that definitions and aims remain complex and that 'the issue of identifying a coherent terminology to describe interprofessional education remains a challenge' (O'Halloran *et al.* 2006: 14). The challenge not only lies in definition and aim but extends into the ability to engage with pedagogical approaches, as if the definition is not clear then it may be difficult to identify the way forward pedagogically for developing curriculum. This can be seen further in this chapter, in the section exploring the pedagogical approaches to emerging curriculum.

Where in the Curriculum Should Interprofessional Learning Take Place?

In the early literature the case was persuasively made for IPL being left until post-qualification. Arguments relating to needing to be confident in one's own professional status, knowledge of practice settings and academic level abounded. However, the growing body of knowledge around the case for collaborative practice has caused the debate about pre- or post-qualifying IPL to virtually disappear. It has been replaced with clarity of focus on pre-qualifying, aided by the support of the Department of Health in establishing four pilot sites in England.

Debate now centres on where in the pre-qualifying curriculum IPL should be centered. Models range from first year, first semester, through all years in isolation through a spiral approach across all years. Early evaluations are eagerly awaited to provide an evidence base that will underpin future models and ways of working relating to curriculum planning.

However, although it is clear that IPL in pre-qualifying curriculum is universally supported, there remains support for the need to ensure that IPL is not lost to post-qualifying education. There is a clear need to continue to embed the learning from pre-qualifying curriculum into the working practice of post-qualifying professionals and it is recognised that the current qualified workforce continues to be representative largely of those professionals who were not exposed to IPL in their pre-qualifying education. Until the predominance of the workforce has had this exposure there will be a need to continue to espouse IPL at post-qualifying level. Furthermore, the models used at post-qualifying level have received much less exposure and tend to concentrate on a shared learning approach, maybe with the exception of the work using a team-based and improvement methodology-based approach as described by Wilcock *et al.* (2003) and by Annandale *et al.* (2000). It is clear that more evaluative work could be undertaken at this level to identify the approaches and pedagogies that may enhance post-qualifying IPL.

Models of Interprofessional Learning in Higher Education Pre-qualifying Health Curriculum

Ways in which IPL are being introduced into curriculum vary but across the literature that shares ways of working there appear to be five clear models emerging:

1. implants as one or more modules into new or existing curriculum;
2. practice placement-based;
3. common curriculum across all professions;
4. e learning in parallel;
5. work based;
6. more than one of the above.

Furthermore, it is clear that whichever of these models is utilised, the approaches may also

- be voluntary or compulsory;
- be extra-curricular or embedded;
- be used to drive new curriculum or parachuted into existing curriculum;
- lump all students within an HEI together or be selective.

Much of this can be explained in relation to the evolution of IPL. It is recognised that getting new ideas and concepts into curriculum already perceived as 'full' with uniprofessional content can challenge existing paradigms. In order to gain credibility, however, there is a need to 'try out' something new, often spearheaded by champions who are at the forefront of new policy drivers and have passion and enthusiasm in the field in which they are trying to gain footage. This is no different for IPL and many early models were only able to gain a foothold by the introduction of voluntary, extra-curricular models of IPL that were bolted on to existing curriculum, sometimes funded through external small project funds, often not funded by anything other than an individual's beliefs and passion for the area.

The difficulties that emerge in gaining consensus of the relevance and value of the work, by the rest of the academic community, then lead to huge barriers in getting from the initial way of working through to an embedded and sustainable model. This will be addressed later in the chapter. However, it is also true to say that without these early pioneer models it is unlikely that the developments that are seen today in England in relation to the variety, depth and adoption of models of IPL that already exist and those that remain in development would never have been achieved. Managing large-scale culture change is recognised as being costly in terms of the time it can take to achieve, and yet there is clarity of recognition of the huge development of IPL now embedded into many of the health professions curriculum in many HEIs, and also identified in the standards set by many of the professional, regulatory and statutory bodies such as the Quality Assurance Agency (QAA), Nursing Midwifery Council (NMC) and Health Professions Council (HPC).

With that in mind it is worth identifying a case study for each model from existing literature.

1. Implants as one or more modules into existing or new curriculum as articulated by the University of the West of England, Bristol

In response to the drive to provide health and social care students with opportunities to learn together to improve interprofessional collaboration, the Faculty of Health and Social Care at the University of the West of England, Bristol, introduced an interprofessional curriculum for its ten pre-qualifying professional programmes in 2000 (Barrett *et al.* 2003).

This model was to implant into a new curriculum three interprofessional modules. Each module was worth 20 credits and one module was implanted into each year of the three year curriculum. The aim of the curriculum was to foster skills for collaborative working through interprofessional groups. Enquiry-based learning, utilising scenarios and underpinned by constructivist learning theories, drove the development. All students learnt in the small groups that reflected the professions offered through the faculty although there was no attempt to manipulate the groups to reflect professional collaboration in practice. A further challenge was the fact that the university had students – in particular nursing students – who had intakes outside the norm and were based on other campuses.

Year one module was classroom based. Year two module utilised a student conference approach and year three delivered online. The module delivery teams were reflective of the diversity of professions in the student groups. Assessment strategies reflect the necessity of engaging the students both individually and in groups, the need to ensure individuality of assessment work and that the assessment contributes to the final award.

In the early days of this new model of working for the faculty (in which the author of this chapter was heavily involved), clear issues emerged including teacher as facilitator, academic staff development to meet this role, understanding of the enormity of resource required to undertake the work, physical resource and space, and co-ordination of the modules as each year unfolded. In addition the challenge to engage those who were neither champions nor convinced of the need for IPL and therefore to change the culture must not be underestimated. Furthermore, the challenge to evaluate in a more robust way than the normal higher education evaluation of modules in order to gain real insight into the impacts and benefits of this way of working was enormous, financially as well as from a methodological perspective.

However, more recent literature (Miers *et al.* 2007) demonstrates that whilst the model is still evolving and some of the issues identified above, such as staff development, remain, students are identifying benefit to their learning from undertaking these modules. In addition, the year three module being online has managed to overcome some of the challenges of multiple campuses and intake times.

2. Practice placement-based as articulated by the TULIP project

The TULIP project is a collaborative venture between Sheffield Hallam University, Nottingham University and NHS Trusts across the East Midlands Strategic Health Authority. The main aim of the project is to develop sustainable models of IPL that will promote and facilitate the professional skills of students through collaborative working within the practice setting. Between the two universities, 13 health and social care pre-qualifying professions are represented.

Between April 2005 and April 2008, eight IPL pilot sites have been operating, incorporating all health and social care communities across the East Midlands Strategic Health Authority region. In order to take the project forward a vital component was the appointment of interprofessional facilitators whose role has been to enable health and social care staff and their students to develop IPL in practice learning. The role of these facilitators has been to identify in practice IPL opportunities that may already exist, and to work with practice staff and students to ensure that students can interact with these opportunities and benefit from them. A further role has been to enable practice staff development with skills to support IPL in practice and to work towards practice adopting an interprofessional philosophy.

In order to underpin this work considerable time was spent developing a capability framework which would underpin the model from a pedagogical perspective. The result of this work has been the Combined Universities Interprofessional Learning Unit (CUILU) interprofessional capability framework (Gordon and Walsh 2005) which is now recognised nationally and being adopted by others to underpin further developments.

In addition, a significant part of the project has been the involvement of service users. In order to achieve this, reference groups of local service users have been set up to inform the project and to become involved in student learning opportunities. A further outcome of the work has been the development of resource packages and training templates for use in practice.

During the lifetime of the project many opportunities have been recognised in practice. Furthermore, the development of specific learning objects such as 'talking heads' has been a feature of the work reflecting the inclusion of service users. In addition, joint working between Coventry University and Sheffield Hallam University in this area has resulted in a combined Centre for Excellence in Interprofessional 'e' teaching and learning.

However, whilst the work of the project has been evident in practice over the time period, the need to ensure sustainability has been a constant concern. The project received funding from the Strategic Health Authority thus enabling the appointment of the facilitators. Whilst it is evident that they have been instrumental in engaging practitioners and students in a number of successful learning opportunities in practice, it remains to be seen whether they have enabled enough culture change for this to be embedded in practitioners once the facilitators are no longer in post. A robust evaluation was carried out between April 2008 and March 2009 and the outcomes of this may give an indication of the longevity and sustainability of the project beyond the funding.

3. Common curriculum across all professions as articulated by the New Generation Project by the University of Southampton

This model was originally devised by the University of Southampton although has since evolved into a collaboration with the University of Portsmouth and the local workforce deanery. Furthermore, this project was recognised by the Department of Health as a vehicle for taking forward common learning in 2002.

The stated aims of the project were to 'introduce students from 11 different health and social care professions to learn together in order to enhance professional collaboration and teamwork skills therefore to improve the quality of care for patients and clients (O'Halloran *et al.* 2006: 12).

This project identified the need to clarify the definition of common learning for all involved and led to the use of the term common learning being perceived as an umbrella term with a range of terms beneath it to describe different facets of the project. For example, IPL was used to identify those sessions which would enable students to learn with, from and about each other and the term learning in common was used to describe opportunities for students to learn the same content as each other but within single profession groups. This understanding was then used to drive the learning, teaching and assessment strategies within the framework. Barr and Ross (2006) identify this model as moving on the existing models, by remodelling much of the uniprofessional content into learning in common and then including intense, interactive small group IPL units across all curriculums.

Key to the project was the need to identify common learning outcomes, both in existing curriculum documents and also as articulated in standards set by QAA for many of the professional groups involved. This led to the identification of what was learning in common, including, for example, IT skills and data analysis skills, as well as areas that were rich for IPL such as understanding diversity, teamworking and service development. The dissemination of this in the literature is resonant with other models where the areas identified above for each aspect of learning resonate with those in models 1 and 4. This is encouraging to note and can give some clarity for those HEIs that are still to engage in this agenda, as the triangulation of this aspect can encourage others to work from this known base rather than having to start from scratch.

Having devised the three IPL units these were then integrated in each year across all the programmes. Kolb's experiential learning paradigm was used to frame the learning model alongside the use of guided discovery learning, collaborative learning and interprofessional learning (Kolb 1984). The key domains, articulated across all units but with differing focus depending on what stage the students are at, are aspects of health and social care practice, experience team working and learning about interprofessional practice. Assessment is then linked to the unit being studied and includes a position paper and an audit as well as a report on practice.

Generically, the units combine both campus and practice based learning, are compulsory, are credit rated and approved by all relevant professional, regulatory and statutory bodies, and contribute fully to the award. Furthermore, many of the issues identified in model 1 such as staff development needs and logistics all apply to this model. However, the model does offer a comprehensive and embedded way of working and, resources permitting, a sustainable one as well. A longitudinal study focusing on the attitudinal and knowledge change in students will provide interesting data for further dissemination and discussion.

4. e learning in parallel as articulated by Coventry University

In 2005 Coventry University validated its interprofessional strategy and framework (in which the author of this chapter was heavily involved in collaboration with the editors of the book, as described in Chapter 6). Three pathways were identified throughout all 11 professional programmes and all were validated in the same week. These were identified as uniprofessional, interprofessional and shared learning. The CAIPE definition was utilised for the interprofessional strand, and the CUILU learning outcomes were adapted to underpin this pathway. The definition for shared learning mimics the discussion at the start of this chapter and also that in model 3, thus identifying common topics whereby students could study to the same learning outcomes and this may or may not happen uni or multiprofessionally.

Problem-based learning was taken as the underpinning pedagogy and included subtypes such as scenario and enquiry-based learning. Web-based patient journeys developed with service users and clients based on a flexible accessible template acted as a catalyst for students to explore patient care in multiple dimensions. In order to manage some of the logistics such as different entry times or differing practice placements, in years two and three, all student work was facilitated in small interprofessional groups. In addition, care was taken to ensure that the patient journey that the student groups were working on was relevant to the students' professions. Therefore this model tried to move away from lumping students together to a more refined way of working designed to reflect the realities of practice.

Furthermore, collaboration with Warwick University Medical School enabled the postgraduate medical students to join with the 11 professional groups at Coventry University to engage with the IPL pathway as part of the small online groups.

Each group was facilitated by an academic member of staff who had undergone the online facilitators training developed by Coventry University. The modules in years two and three carried 20 credits each, were compulsory, managed on a pass/fail basis and therefore contributed to the final award. Assessment was clearly linked to the online contribution made by each student and this proved crucial in ensuring that the students engaged although provoked a steep learning curve for the first cohort of students, some of whom failed as a result on non-engagement. Interestingly, whilst this was clearly upsetting for students, it was even more upsetting for staff, particularly those who were not engaging with the interprofessional agenda and had not 'heard' the message about its role in the new curriculum.

Similarly to others though, this model again brought with it issues relating to workload capacity and staff development. In addition, the logistics of developing the online facilities, the complexity of enabling students and academic staff from a neighbouring university to enrol as students in order to gain access to the online learning environment, and the management of the student groups online must not be underestimated. However, the use of service users to develop the patient journeys and the opportunity to manage this from any computer wherever you were, which in terms of the issues surrounding complex curriculum and student practice placements, were seen as a bonus. This model is now nearing its first cohort to exit and dissemination of evaluation results will be eagerly awaited.

5. Work based learning as articulated by the University of Derby

Barr and Ross (2006) suggest that work based initiatives in IPL are now mainly being used by universities wanting to retain a foothold in post-qualifying education. Whilst not disagreeing that this focus seems appropriate, the University of Derby has recently articulated a model of IPL that, whilst employing the CAIPE definition, has moved beyond having this as the focus and, in partnership with the NHS Institute of Innovation and Improvement, has rooted its IPL in skills development and improvement methodology and practice.

The use of 'laboratories' to engage students in IPL is not new. However, at the University of Derby the interpretation of laboratories goes beyond the traditional skills labs used for health, to include a crime scene house, a law court and other forensic arenas. For example, health and social care and law students in year two of their curriculum are exposed to a court room scenario. The law students get the opportunity to act as examiner-in-chief and the health and social care students the opportunity to act as an expert witness. Whilst the emphasis is on developing skills in relation to care of vulnerable adults and preparing statements for court, an additional aim is to offer work in an interprofessional context. Student feedback identifies that although the emphasis appears to be on skill acquisition, the opportunity to learn with, from and about each other is also articulated well.

Health and social care students in year three of their programme are currently being introduced to healthcare improvement methodologies whilst on campus and gaining experience of ways of working such as process mapping. They are then enabled to go out into practice in groups of five or six to work with an improvement facilitator on an issue identified by that facilitator relevant to the area of practice. Facilitators may be qualified health and social care staff, may be managers and include acute and primary care areas and general practices. In practice students investigate the issue and use the new tools they have been exposed to in order to provide the practice area with a report with suggestions for improvement. To date, these reports have provided creative solutions and resulted in, for example, a reduction in, inpatient stays for toe surgery. The value to the students in being able to influence and change practice is hugely motivating, and NHS trusts are articulating the improvement to patient care.

This model was initially developed as a project but has now been embedded into five professional curriculums and has provoked the development of the faculty's interprofessional strategy.

The emphasis in this model is not relayed to the students as learning with, from and about each other. Whilst the CUILU outcomes are embedded in modules, the emphasis is on the focus of skill acquisition or improvement processes. The IPL is therefore acquired more through process rather than declaration and has benefited from a more work-based approach giving relevance to the work in hand and enabling the students to work out for themselves the benefit of interprofessional teamwork and collaborative working.

The modules attract credit, are compulsory and contribute to the award. Assessment is undertaken through contribution to a portfolio. Issues arising from this way of working have included staff development, but rather than focusing on facilitation of IPL have moved to focusing on facilitation of improvement methodology. A benefit has been the ability to access general practice for student experience and the addition of learning for the practice improvement facilitators. Desire to facilitate is now outstripping demand by student groups and improvement to patient care is being evaluated robustly as part of the project.

6. Model 6 – more than one of the above

In reality many of the models articulated above are not pure models and engage in a pick and mix approach to facilitate their IPL agendas. What has been portrayed here is an outline of where the model is largely as identified in the hope that the reader is enabled to gain an insight into the key ways of working and benefits and challenges to the model. Each of the institutions identified either has or indicates that it will be publishing material related to its model and the reader is encouraged to look out for this and engage with the material as appropriate.

Pedagogy to Support Learning, Teaching and Assessment in Interprofessional Learning

A pedagogical approach to the theoretical underpinning is described in the majority of case study models articulated in the section above. Similarities and differences are apparent and it is important to question these in order identify commonality and whether this is underpinned by evidence so that future IPL models can learn from current experience. Three common areas appear – the use of experiential learning, the use of case study/scenario/patient journeys and the use of small groups.

Experiential learning

Kolb's (1984) experiential learning cycle is clearly articulated as an underpinning feature in the University of Southampton model, with other models articulating a preference for experiential learning without necessarily citing Kolb.

Kolb's experiential learning theory describes the sort of learning undertaken by students who are given a chance to acquire and apply knowledge, skills and feelings in an immediate and relevant setting. Experiential learning thus involves a direct encounter with the phenomena being studied rather than merely thinking about the encounter, or only considering the possibility of doing something about it. This sort of learning is sponsored by an institution and sits well with programmes for professions where both theory and practice based learning experiences are offered. Kolb and Fry (1975) argue that the learning cycle can begin at any one of the four points of their cycle – and that it should really be approached as a continuous spiral. However, it is suggested that the learning process often begins with a person carrying out a particular action and then seeing the effect of the action in this situation. Following this, the second step is to understand these effects in the particular instance so that if the same action was taken in the same circumstances it would be possible to anticipate what would follow from the action. In this pattern the third step would be understanding the general principle under which the particular instance falls. The relevance for this in relation to IPL cannot be ignored, offering students the opportunity to experience the new phenomena, understand the effects of this way of working and then move to a position whereby the student can transfer the principles of the learning into multiple situations over time.

However, whilst there is good support for Kolb's theory and indeed further variants of it (Honey and Mumford 1982) there are issues with it as a model if used in the singular.

Boud (1995) argues that it pays insufficient attention to the process of reflection so that whilst it may be useful in assisting us in planning learning activities and in helping us to check simply that learners can be effectively engaged, it does not help to uncover the elements of reflection itself.

Second, the model takes very little account of different cultural experiences/conditions (Anderson 1988). The inventory has also been used within a fairly limited range of cultures (an important consideration if we approach learning as situated, i.e. affected by environments). As Anderson (1988, cited in Tennant 1997) highlights, there is a need to take account of differences in cognitive and communication styles that are culturally based. Here we need to attend to different models of selfhood – and the extent to which these may differ from the 'western' assumptions that underpin the Kolb and Fry model.

Third, the idea of stages or steps does not sit well with the reality of thinking. There is a problem here – that of sequence. As Dewey (1933) has said in relation to reflection a number of processes can occur at once, stages can be jumped. This way of presenting things is rather too neat and is simplistic.

Fourth, empirical support for the model is weak (Jarvis 1987; Tennant 1997). The initial research base was small, and there have only been a limited number of studies that have sought to test or explore the model (such as Jarvis 1987). Furthermore, the learning style inventory 'has no capacity to measure the degree of integration of learning styles' (Tennant 1997: 92).

Finally, the relationship of learning processes to knowledge is problematic. As Jarvis (1987) again points out, Kolb is able to show that learning and knowledge are intimately related. However, Kolb does not really explore the nature of knowledge in any depth and therefore it could be argued that his model does not really grasp different ways of knowing. For example, Kolb focuses on processes in the individual mind, rather than seeing learning as situated. Furthermore, in Kolb's model learning is concerned with the production of knowledge. 'Knowledge results from the combination of grasping experience and transforming it' (Kolb 1984: 41) whereas in IPL we may want the focus to be on informed and committed action.

Given these problems, academics are advised to take some care when using Kolb's learning cycle. However, as Tennant (1997: 92) points out, the model provides an excellent framework for planning teaching and learning activities and it can be usefully employed as a guide for enabling experience and building on that experience in professional education.

Constructivist learning theories

The term refers to the idea that learners construct knowledge for themselves – each learner individually (and socially) constructs meaning – as he or she learns. If the belief is that learning consists of individuals' constructed meanings then it is important that we consider how this may impact onto the way of working in relation to IPL.

Clear principles of constructivist learning theories include the following:

- Learning needs to be identified as an active process in which the learner uses sensory input and constructs meaning out of it. Therefore activities need to engage the learner in doing something so that learning is not the passive acceptance of knowledge which exists 'out there'.
- People learn to learn as they learn: learning consists both of constructing meaning and constructing systems of meaning. For example, if we learn the chronology of dates of a series of historical events, we are simultaneously learning the meaning of a chronology. Each meaning we construct makes us better able to give meaning to other sensations which can fit a similar pattern.
- The crucial action of constructing meaning is mental: it happens in the mind. Physical actions, hands-on experience may be necessary for learning, especially for children, but it is not sufficient; we need to provide activities which engage the mind as well as the hands.
- Learning involves language: the language we use influences learning. Therefore the way in which we interact and the language used in materials and interactions influences whether individuals are able to construct meaning or not.
- Learning is a social activity: therefore our learning is intimately associated with our connection with other human beings, for example, our teachers and our peers. Therefore education based on this theory must recognise the social aspect of learning and uses conversation, interaction with others, and the application of knowledge as an integral aspect of learning.
- Learning is contextual: we do not learn isolated facts and theories in some abstract ethereal land of the mind separate from the rest of our lives: we learn in relationship to what else we know, what we believe,

our prejudices and our fears. On reflection, it becomes clear that this point is actually a corollary of the idea that learning is active and social. We cannot divorce our learning from our lives.

- One needs knowledge to learn: it is not possible to assimilate new knowledge without having some structure developed from previous knowledge to build on. The more we know, the more we can learn. Therefore any effort to teach must be connected to the state of the learner, must provide a path into the subject for the learner based on that learner's previous knowledge. In the UWE model the fact that it was the final year module that was based on this theory could be argued to be consistent with this point as previous IPL in years one and two using other theories would have provided previous knowledge for the learners to build on.

- It takes time to learn: learning is not instantaneous. For significant learning we need to revisit ideas, ponder them, try them out, play with them and use them. This cannot happen in 5–10 minutes. Therefore the span of planned interprofessional activity both in one session and over time becomes important.

- Motivation is a key component in learning. Not only is it the case that motivation helps learning, it is essential for learning. Therefore unless we know why the knowledge may be useful we may not gain enough motivation to ensure learning. This may resonate with early evaluations of IPL within first year pre-qualifying curriculum which suggested that learners found the learning difficult to ascribe meaning to, probably due to lack of professional knowledge and understanding and therefore identified lack of motivation in relation to the interprofessional component of their programme of study.

As Miers *et al.* (2007) identify, the choice of this as a learning theory offered the opportunity to add to the exploration of the range of theories that may inform and explain effective IPL. Constructivist learning theory does seem to offer academics not only a theoretical approach to learning but promotes ways of learning, teaching and assessment that have some resonance with current models of IPL to date.

Co-operative learning

D'Eon (2005) suggests that co-operative learning can also offer a way of working for IPL. Co-operative learning uses experiential learning but also works on the use of five elements which are listed in Box 3.1.

Box 3.1 Five Elements of Co-Operative Learning

1. Mutual interdependence;
2. Face-to-face promotive interaction;
3. Individual accountability;
4. Interpersonal and small group skills and group processing;
5. Use of the experiential learning cycle.

The literature identifies that co-operative learning is very effective in promoting learning to work in teams (Crosby and Hesketh 2004).

For IPL particularly if this aim is clearly articulated in the programme, this can offer a way of structuring the learning and teaching. However, whilst elements 1, 3 and 4 are often described as being present, this way of working does not work for some forms of e learning, which may not promote at present the use of web cams or live classroom and may also be asynchronous.

Bourdieu's theory of habitus (Bourdieu 1977, 1990)

Many papers identify that the main barrier to interprofessional working lies in the fact that professional identities compete rather than work together on the common focus of service delivery.

Our professional identity is developed through a socialisation process and this gives us the template by which our behaviour and values are determined. Bourdieu calls this template 'habitus' and he suggests that this gives rise to the internalised structures that people use to classify themselves and others. Bourdieu also identifies that habitus is the cognitive map that an individual calls upon to make socially acceptable decisions.

In health and social care professional education, individuals conform to their respective professional standards and competencies thus enabling each professional group to identify their unique role both as an individual and in relation to their profession and leading to a sense of belonging or, as Giddens terms it, 'ontological security'. We see this in the professional silos that are described and it is this habitus that leads to the strengthening of professional boundaries.

Using habitus as a theory suggests that the objective of IPL is to enable different professionals to understand each other's cognitive map and to attempt to establish an interprofessional habitus, that is, one shared by different professionals. In using this theory to underpin

IPL there are several key messages (Box 3.2) that can be used to form the basis for learning using habitus:

Box 3.2 Key Messages for IPL Based on Theory of Habitus

1. Flexibility of professional habitus. There is always scope for change, and learning can promote a new more interprofessional habitus through work-based initiatives and the use of novel situations that require an individual to think and react in new ways.
2. Modelling of norms. If we want to see an interprofessional habitus develop then we need to engage with those modelling this in practice which includes professionals working across boundaries and also service users. If the overarching goal is to entertain a patient-led agenda and patients are clear that working with one professional group is not the norm then this becomes a powerful catalyst for changing habitus. Therefore the way in which IPL is integrated into practice becomes important if a new interprofessional habitus is to be promoted.
3. Generational change needs to occur. If new ways of being are not to be stifled by existing ways of working then education not only needs to offer a new habitus to pre-qualifying students but at the same time needs to develop this new habitus in the existing workforce, thus increasing the rate of change so that a new norm is established more quickly than may otherwise have been possible.

As a way of thinking, habitus is complex but worth pursuing and may be partially seen in the University of Derby model, whereby inter-professional learning is engaging both pre-qualifying students and the existing workforce, using a service user–led agenda to improve care, and challenges the individual professional norms to move towards a more interprofessional habitus over time.

Whilst there are other theories in the literature those described above demonstrate that no one theory is currently recognised as the right one for IPL. It is also recognised that most of the models outlined are using a mix of pedagogies to inform their curriculum development, and that experiential learning seems to be involved in some way, shape or form.

However, what is noteworthy is that nearly all the models scrutinised identify the use of scenarios/cases/patient journeys developed from service users either directly or indirectly.

As identified in the discussion regarding habitus, the patient-led agenda is clearly driving the current NHS policy and strategy. This can be seen in patient choice, the plethora of Web sites on which patient stories are available, for example, the genetics education centre Web site, the DIPEX Web site and in learning objects being developed for IPL. The use of service users is increasing in educational programmes and often linked to interprofessional strategies in HEIs.

Alongside this it was clear that all models worked with small groups of students, whether online or face to face, whether campus based or practice based. Whilst this gives rise to huge implications on workload and resource availability, there seems to be consensus that IPL benefits from this as a way of working, although it must be recognised that the concept of small group ranges from 6 to 15, probably in part dependent on the number of students at any one time in the institution and therefore number of academic staff available. Those models that have managed this most successfully have engaged in a partnership with practice to facilitate the groups thus maximising the availability of facilitators and encouraging the partnership in educational delivery. This appears to have been most successful in those models where at least part of the delivery is practice based, models 3 and 5 in particular.

It could therefore be suggested that the use of service users and clients to share their stories and the use of small groups are in some way integral to successful IPL. However, the challenges to developing these ways of working are considerable and lead to an exploration in the final section of this chapter.

Mainstreaming/integration and sustainability of interprofessional learning

Interprofessional learning has been gradually creeping into professional education over the last three decades and is now being mainstreamed in a way that would not have been thought possible even five years ago. However, whilst policy has driven the engagement with interprofessional agendas, we are in danger of seeing this being overlaid by competing agendas such as the modernising of the NHS and the modernisation of health and social care careers and therefore professional education systems. It is therefore imperative that we continue to identify the purpose and meaning of IPL and also reconcile this to the competing agendas if further progress is to be made. Barr and Ross (2006) outline this eloquently in their position paper.

Of more concern, however, is the sustainability of IPL. Most of the literature and certainly author experience identify the many challenges that are faced in relation to setting up IPL in the first place. These include, but are not exhaustive of (Box 3.3):

Box 3.3 Challenges to Sustainability

- moving from a staff base of few champions to an integration of IPL across faculty, to include practitioners as well as academics;
- the huge human resource needed to maintain small group ways of working;
- the funds and skills required to develop learning objects that are often e-based and service user-based;
- the funds and skills required to develop and implement e-based models of IPL;
- physical resource to host multiple small groups;
- time for innovation in learning, teaching and assessment;
- barriers between interprofessional faculty;
- tensions between competing demands on curriculum time in relation to uniprofessional versus interprofessional content.

For many of the models outlined above there is clear identification of innovative ways of working, much of which has been funded by faculty resource that is not reflected in benchmark pricing or Higher Education Funding Council for England (HEFCE) core funding. If we are to have a chance of continuing to sustain and develop in innovative ways then this has to be rectified. Furthermore, any cuts in resources as seen more recently in the reduction of contract numbers in an unplanned way across England can compromise the ability to run small groups effectively, a clear challenge to a way of working that seems to be linked to successful outcomes of IPL.

To date, professional, statutory and regulatory bodies have begun to play their part in ensuring that IPL is sustained by including IPL in standards and benchmark statements. However, with the review of the number and function of the regulatory bodies there is a chance that this may be weakened and this could contribute to a lack of sustainability over time.

Other more local factors could also contribute to a lack of sustainability. It is clear that those institutions that have been successful have in part managed this due to champions and senior management support and involvement. However, relying on champions is not the way forward and many HEIs have invested in developing faculty. However, if this is not sustained and included in induction for new staff and teaching programmes then again sustainability is questionable, as senior managers move on and support wanes or enthusiasm wanes amongst faculty with no succession planning in place.

It is also recognised that there are more and more competing claims on faculty workload to include income generation, research and publication. Whilst these are not inherently bad they could become the cause of a lack of innovation in relation to future developments in IPL.

Finally, it is recognised that HEIs must ensure engagement with and application to practice if IPL is to be both meaningful and sustainable in the long term.

Whilst the above dialogue could be seen as pessimistic it is hoped that this will promote clarity around the need to engage with current agendas and to succession plan to safeguard the future of IPL for future health and social care professionals to contribute to the improvement of patient/client care.

Conclusion

This chapter has set out to explore models, pedagogies and realities in relation to IPL in higher education. It is hoped that this exploration will be of benefit to those planning to engage in IPL in the future. However, whilst ideals have been offered it is recognised that curriculum design is always a compromise between the educational ideal, the teaching and learning resources available and what will work in the local context (O'Halloran *et al.* 2006: 26). With that in mind we are to be encouraged to try to balance these competing demands as we seek to learn from the experience of others and continue to innovate in IPL practice.

References

Anderson, J.A. (1988). Cognitive styles and multicultural populations. *Journal of Teacher Education*, 39 (1): 2–9.

Annandale, S.J., S. McCann, H. Nattrass, S.R. de Bere, S. Williams and D. Evans. (2000). Achieving health improvements through interprofessional learning in south west England. *Journal of Interprofessional Care*, 14: 161–179.

Barr, H. (2002). *Interprofessional Education: Today, Yesterday and Tomorrow*. London: LTSN Health Sciences and Practice.

Barr, H. and F. Ross. (2006). Mainstreaming interprofessional education in the United Kingdom: A position paper. *Journal of Interprofessional Care*, 20 (2): 96–104.

Barrett, G., R. Greenwood and K. Ross. (2003). Integrating interprofessional education into 10 health and social care programmes. *Journal of Interprofessional Care*, 17 (3): 293–301.

Boud, D. (1995). *Enhancing Learning Through Self Assessment*. London: Kogan Page.

Bourdieu, P. (1977). *Outline of a Theory of Practice*. Cambridge: Cambridge University Press.

Bourdieu, P. (1990). *The Logic of Practice*. Standford, CA: Standford University Press.

CAIPE (1997). Interprofessional education – A definition. *CAIPE Bulletin*, 13, 19. London: Centre for the Advancement of Interprofessional Education.

Crosby, J.R. and E.A. Hesketh. (2004). Developing the teaching instinct 11: Small group learning. *Medical Teacher*, 26 (1): 16–19.

D'Eon, M. (2005). A blue print for Interprofessional learning. *Journal of Interprofessional Care*, May, 19 (1): 49–59.

Department of Health. (2001). *A Health Service for All the Talents: Developing the NHS Workforce*. London: Department of Health.

Dewey, J. (1933). *How We Think: A Restatement of the Relation of Reflective Thinking to the Educative Process*. Boston: DC Heath and Company.

Gordon, F. and C. Walsh. (2005). A framework for interprofessional capability: Developing students of health and social care as collaborative workers. *Journal of Integrated Care*, 13 (3): 26–33.

Honey, P. and A. Mumford. (1982). *Manual of Learning Styles*. London: P. Henry.

Jarvis, P. (1987). *Adult Learning in the Social Context*. London: Croom Helm.

Kolb, D. and R. Fry. (1975). Toward an applied theory of experimental learning. In C. Cooper (ed.) *Theories of Group Process*. London: John Wiley.

Kolb, D.A. (1984). *Experiential Learning: Experience as the Source of Learning and Development*. Englewood Cliffs, NH: Prentice-Hall.

Miers, M.E., B.A. Clarke, K.C. Pollard, C.E. Rickarby, J. Thomas and A. Turtle. (2007). Online interprofessional learning: The student experience. *Journal of Interprofessional Care*, 21(5), 529–542.

Miller, C., M. Freeman and N. Ross. (2001). *Interprofessional Practice in Health and Social Care: Challenging the Shared Learning Agenda*. London: Arnold.

O'Halloran, C., S. Hean, D. Humphris and J. Macleod-Clark. (2006). Developing common learning: The New Generation Project undergraduate curriculum model. *Journal of Interprofessional Care*, 20: 12–28.

Tennant, M. (1997). *Psychology and Adult Learning*, 2nd edn. London: Routledge.

Wilcock, P., C. Campion-Smith and S. Elston. (2003). *Practice Professional Development Planning: A Guide for Primary Care*. Oxford: Radcliffe Medical Press.

World Health Organisation. (1987). *Learning Together to Work Together for Health*. Report of a WHO Study Group on Multiprofessional Education of Health Personnel: The Team Approach, Technical Report Series 769. Geneva: World Health Organisation.

Zwarenstein, M., S. H. Reeves, H. Hammick, I. Koppel and J. Atkins. (2000) Interprofessional education: Effects on professional practice and health care outcomes (Cochrane Review). *The Cochrane Library*. Chichester: John Wiley & Sons, Ltd.

4

Interprofessional Capability as an Aim of Student Learning

Frances Gordon

Introduction

This chapter is based on work undertaken previously by the Combined Universities Interprofessional Learning Unit (CUILU),[1] and draws on findings and project work concerned with identifying what students need to learn, in order to become capable of effective collaborative practice in changing health and social care arenas. The Interprofessional Capability Framework will be discussed as a tool for guiding and assessing student learning, and utilising the Framework, issues around how education for interprofessional capability has been developed will be described.

Contemporary health and social care practice demands that practitioners are developed in skills of collaboration. Collaboration, as an aim of working practices, has arisen from a slow burn of discontent expressed by the users of services and, in recent decades in the UK, escalated by the occurrence of a number of high profile medico-legal disasters. Subsequent public enquiries identified failure of individuals and agencies to effectively communicate and work in an integrated way, as factors in what went wrong. See, for example, the Bristol Enquiry Final Report (Kennedy, 2001) and the Victoria Climbié Report (Laming, 2003).

Attempts to change practice have been made partly due to professional recognition that traditional ways of working are failing those we care for. Perhaps a stronger driver is the implementation of policy initiatives that are intended to support developments that focus on the need to centre provision on the needs of service users and their informal carers, rather than services being designed in the ways most convenient for the organisation to operate them. These initiatives have been prolific over recent years and impetus that gathered pace during the first decade of the millennium was encouraged by documents such as *The NHS Plan* (DH, 2000) and the Expert Patient (DH, 2002). The intention of this agenda to modernise health and social care services was to provide an integrated service for service users and their carers, a central recognition being that professionals within and across services require to work together effectively (DH, 1997, 1999, 2001). This predisposes a notion that practitioners, graduating from health and social care professional courses, are required to be competent in skills of collaboration to enable them to function effectively as the modernisation agenda drives towards the development of increasingly integrated services.

Preparing interprofessionally capable practitioners

Much of the reporting about interprofessional education (IPE) has focused on relatively small-scale interventions, involving a limited range of professions and seldom during undergraduate education and training (Freeth *et al.*, 2002). Undergraduate IPE in health and social care is notoriously difficult to implement systematically on a wider scale, due to logistical and other barriers (CIPeL, 2006).[2] However, IPE in terms of students learning *with, from and about each other* (Barr, 2002) is gaining ground in the undergraduate curricula of many institutions. This raises questions of exactly what is it that students are required to learn in these instances. Barr's proposals around learning with, from and about give some helpful direction, and knowing more about the roles and attributes of the other professions contributing to the care of service users underpins being able to work with them. However, this chapter aims to add more detail, in the articulation of what students require to learn, in order to become effective interprofessional practitioners.

Barr (2002) has argued that capability, rather than competence, better recognises the many-layered and multiple processes that professionals are expected to perform. This is in keeping with Wilson and Holt's (2001) argument that concentrating only on 'competence' may not be sufficient to prepare practitioners to respond effectively to the challenge of working in contemporary health and social care. This suggests that the complexity of practice isn't fully taken into account by the concept of 'competence' because many conceptualisations of competence focus on the performance of a task (Heron and Murray, 2004). Conversely, it was suggested over a decade ago by Hagar and Gonezi (1996) that a too narrow view of competence is often accepted uncritically, and that a richer conceptualisation is possible, although this does seem to defeat its own argument by suggesting additional richness is required. There is a body of literature that explores every conceivable definition, and understanding of competence and capability, as such this argument continues to rage. However, the work described in this chapter is based upon an interpretation of Fraser and Greenhalgh's (2001) definition of capability. This being one where competence is incorporated, and the process of being able to successfully undertake a 'task' is seen as important, and reflected in what will be described later. However, although a form of competence is included in the Capability Framework as a learning level, this is extended in capability to ensure an integrated application of knowledge where the student or practitioner can adapt to change, develop new behaviours and continue to improve performance. This includes the demonstration of tasks, the performance of which evolves as part of complex, changing practice.

The CUILU Interprofessional Capability Framework draws on the work of the Sainsbury Centre for Mental Health (SCMH) – *The Capable Practitioner*. The learning outcomes contained in the Interprofessional Capability Framework are incremental, intended to guide student practice, and stated in terms of learning achievements leading to 'capability', a term defined by the SCMH report (2001: 2) as having the following dimensions (Box 4.1):

Box 4.1 Learning Achievements Leading to 'Capability'

- A performance component which identifies 'what people need to possess' and 'what they need to achieve' in the workplace;
- An ethical component that is concerned with integrating a knowledge of culture, values and social awareness into professional practice;
- A component that emphasises reflective practice in action;
- The capability to effectively implement evidence-based interventions in the service configurations of a modern mental health system;
- A commitment to working with new models of professional practice and responsibility for lifelong learning.

Taking into account the above, the Interprofessional Capability Framework is concerned not only with *doing*, as in its performance and implementation components, but also with *knowing* and *being*, as seen in its ethical reflection and lifelong learner dimensions. The Framework was developed with the student practitioner in mind, although the validation processes of the Framework reported elsewhere (Gordon *et al.*, 2006) illuminated self-assessed learning needs among qualified staff. Use of the Framework should be based on an assumption that as adult learners, students will bring to the workplace previous knowledge, and will actively engage with what they need to learn in order to meet their specific learning needs (Knowles, 1990). Achievement of the incremental steps, leading to capability, is therefore underpinned by theoretical concepts derived from campus-based study, informed by practice experience, and supported by the knowledge and expertise of practice based educators.

Determining that students of health and social care should be not only competent, but extend to capable interprofessional workers is, however, just the beginning of the issue. What the required competencies and capabilities articulate is an important issue, as when taken as a whole the Framework may define interprofessional practice. This is an interesting point, in that although strategies that may facilitate interprofessional learning have been described quite extensively in the literature, the term 'interprofessional working' itself is poorly understood, and little work is reported regarding learning the processes of interprofessional *practice* (McCray, 2003). This is reflected by the practices of deriving intuitively and/or through common sense considerations learning outcomes labelled as interprofessional. At times, the learning is planned to address 'common' issues that all students need to learn such as ethical theory, research approaches or even anatomy and physiology – although the latter is thankfully less common. Other concepts frequently addressed under the interprofessional rubric are communication skills, team structures and processes and shared decision-making.

What the CUILU team set out to do was to provide students and their educational facilitators with more systematically derived learning outcomes in terms of stated competencies and capabilities. These statements were formulated with the aim of making clear what students needed to learn in order to become collaborative workers.

The development of the Interprofessional Capability Framework has been described elsewhere (Gordon and Walsh, 2005; Walsh *et al.*, 2005), but in summary the CUILU team aimed to derive learning outcomes that reflected the complexity of interprofessional working in terms of capability, and show the incremental learning that would lead to the capability. It was important that these could be shown to be relevant to all professional groups. If the tenets of interprofessional learning were to be met – '... when two or more professions learn with, from and about each other in order to improve collaboration and the quality of care' (Barr, 2002) – it seemed obvious that students learning together needed to be working towards the same outcomes. It also seemed obvious that these outcomes should in some way contribute to the development of collaborative skills. The Higher Education Quality Assurance Agency (QAA, 2000, 2001, 2002) benchmark statements relating to the undergraduate programmes of medicine, dentistry and the professions allied to medicine including nursing, midwifery and social work were used as a source for generating the capabilities required for undertaking interprofessional practice.

Recognising that the concept of interprofessional practice or working was poorly defined (McCray, 2003), the team worked to clarify their ideas through the literature and by drawing on collective experience in practice and education. Hall and Weaver's (2001) work was a useful starting point. They differentiate between *multidisciplinary* working, where care is underpinned by parallel but independent contributions based on particular expertise; *interdisciplinary working* where, whilst preserving specialised functions, there is close communication and supported contributions allowing holistic management of the patient's health needs; and *transdisciplinary* working where roles and functions overlap, indicating that colleagues must be familiar with the concepts and approaches of each other's professional roles.

Rushmer's (2005) work, however, calls for caution in situations where professions work closely together, raising the potential for conflict and lack of cohesive care if different groups carry out similar practices without consultation and communication. In her description of working in a fully integrated way – which she describes as successful interprofessional working – the overlaps in practice between professions are agreed through negotiation and are therefore not intrusive or threatening.

Barr's (2002: 6) work is also helpful in that he makes the distinction between multiprofessional education as 'occasions when two or more professions learn side by side for whatever reason' and IPE as 'occasions when two or more professions learn from and about each other to improve collaboration and quality of care'. Utilising insights from their own practice, and by drawing on Hall and Weaver's work, and on Barr's definitions, the team proposed that interprofessional working is defined by drawing together the descriptions of interdisciplinary and transdisciplinary working. Interprofessional working may be described as

A process that places the patient/service user at the centre of the activity, where individual contributions of the care team are collaborative in nature and where roles and functions may overlap, in order to provide the best possible care for the individual and his or her carers.

(Gordon and Ward, 2005)

This definition provided a sensitising theoretical thread when analysing the QAA benchmarks. The benchmarks were interrogated to isolate those statements, which appeared in some form, across all subject benchmarks and underpinned what the team believed interprofessional practice to be. Once these had been isolated, further work was done to categorise them into domains. These were ethical practice, knowledge in practice, interprofessional working and reflection.

One advantage of the approach taken is that any notion of interprofessional learning being either irrelevant or an optional component of student learning can be dispelled by the fact that the outcomes contained within the Framework can be tracked back to participating students' programme-specific quality benchmarks.

The Interprofessional Capability Framework

The Framework in its entirety can be accessed at www.shef.ac.uk/cuilu. Presented below are the 16 capabilities derived through the analysis of the QAA benchmark statements. The capabilities are grouped into the categorical domains of ethical practice, knowledge in practice, interprofessional working and reflection (Boxes 4.2–4.5).

Box 4.2 The Interprofessional Capability Framework – Capabilities of Ethical Practice Domain

Domain: Ethical Practice

Capability

1. The interprofessional team member continually develops, promotes and practises understanding and respect for others' cultures, values and belief systems.

2. The interprofessional team member interacts within the health and social care practice community to consistently promote and support patient/user participation and autonomy, on the basis of informed decision-making and exercise of choice.
3. The interprofessional team member consistently ensures an interprofessional approach to the exercise of duty of care, within a legal and ethical framework.
4. The interprofessional team member critically evaluates policy and practice in the context of

   • patient/client-focused care
   • the changing role boundaries that inform the nature of the interprofessional team
   • making recommendations to influence developments to improve the quality of service/care for patients/clients of the service.

Box 4.3 The Interprofessional Capability Framework – Capabilities of Knowledge in Practice Domain

Domain: Knowledge in Practice

Capability

5. The interprofessional team member has an integrated understanding of the legal frameworks and statutory and regulatory requirements of the professions that make up the practice team.
6. The interprofessional team member exercises a critical understanding of team structures and effective team functioning, through knowledge of group dynamics and professional roles of all team members.
7. The interprofessional team member maintains and develops a critical understanding of the requirements and non-judgemental and anti-discriminatory practice in order to effectively participate in care management decisions.

Box 4.4 The Interprofessional Capability Framework – Capabilities of Interprofessional Working Domain

Domain: Interprofessional Working

Capability

8. The interprofessional team member is able to lead or participate in interprofessional team and wider inter-agency work, to ensure a responsive and integrated approach to care/service management that is focused on the needs of the patient/client.

Box 4.4 (Continued)

9. The interprofessional team member implements an integrated assessment and plan of care/service in partnership with the patient/client, remaining responsive to the dynamic needs of care/service requirements.
10. The interprofessional team member consistently communicates sensitively in a responsive and responsible manner, demonstrating effective interpersonal skills in the context of patient/client-focused care.
11. The interprofessional team member shares uniprofessional knowledge with the team in ways that contribute to and enhances service provision.
12. The interprofessional team member provides a co-mentoring role to peers of own or other professions in order to enhance service provision and personal and professional development.

Box 4.5 The Interprofessional Capability Framework – Capabilities of the Reflection Domain

Domain: Reflection

Capability

13. The interprofessional team member utilises reflective processes in order to work in partnership with patients and colleagues, ensuring a patient/client focused, and integrated care/service provision.
14. The interprofessional team member utilises a reciprocal process of reflection and supervision to support the continual development of the interprofessional team.
15. The interprofessional team member responds to the needs of the service by utilising problem-solving approaches and evidence-based practice to identify and anticipate future changes in interprofessional team role.
16. The interprofessional team member addresses professional development and lifelong learning needs in the interests of personal, professional and organisational/service development.

Validating the Framework

Devising a Framework is only the first step in its production. Evaluating how it would work in practice is a necessary requirement before it can be recommended for use. The Framework underwent a validation process in the National Health Service (NHS) practice areas, used as pilot sites by the CUILU project (Gordon *et al.*, 2006). These areas were selected against specified criteria and were considered to be environments that offered rich interprofessional learning opportunities to students (Gordon *et al.*, 2004).

Strategies to validate the Framework involved qualitative interviews with students on placement ($n = 39$), in the beacon sites, and the practitioners who supported them ($n = 22$). One purpose of the interviews was to 'test' the conceptual domains within the Framework. This aspect was addressed by both practitioners and students who were given the Framework, as a reference point throughout the students' practice placements. The participants were asked to reflect on whether and how the capabilities could be achieved in their practice area, thus considering their 'fit' with how interprofessional working was perceived. The views of the participants, on whether they considered the capabilities in the Framework were relevant to and appropriate for their own profession, were also explored. Due to greater experience, and their roles in supporting students of other professions, the practitioners were also asked to comment on whether they felt any of the capabilities were not appropriate to any of the professions. Students were also asked to self-assess their performance against the Framework at the end of their placement, and practitioners were also asked to use the Framework to assess the students they had supervised.

The full report of the validation study can be accessed in the CUILU final report (Gordon *et al.*, 2006). However, the findings of the evaluation processes highlighted a number of key points and are replicated below:

- **The Framework provides a statement of what students need to learn**

    The capabilities and learning outcomes contained in the Framework were recognised as appropriate and relevant to the participants' own and other professions' learning. This supports the use of the Framework as providing learning outcomes that are common to and relevant for all students.

- **The Framework draws attention to learning opportunities that promote interprofessional working**

    The learning outcomes within the Framework sensitise its users to interprofessional aspects of the learning opportunities available in the practice context. This carries the potential for developing the interprofessional focus of the practice context by extending consideration of a learning opportunity, as a topic to be learned, such as a clinical skill, to a wider view of the topic as an interprofessional and collaborative working issue relevant to interprofessional learning.

- ## Service organisation can limit interprofessional learning

  Although the beacon sites were recognised as areas where interprofessional working took place, the success in facilitating interprofessional learning for students seemed to be positively related to how integrated both the service organisation and students' support in the beacon sites were. Where barriers to organising interprofessional learning seem to be in operation, it was not because of lack of learning opportunities, but a function of the students' experience being managed in profession-specific contexts. This resulted in students learning, in the same setting, in isolation from each other. Non-integrated structures within the organisation, communication difficulties between professions both in practice and in the university context, and educational funding stream issues were also cited as reasons for not integrating student learning fully.

- ## The Framework's potential to advance interprofessional practice

  When organising learning opportunities across professions for students, learning objectives tend to be set at a level that the 'visiting' student could reasonably achieve, and will be at a lower level than their profession-specific objectives. This is because the student could not be expected to have proficiency in another profession's skills or knowledge. Such objectives, however, do not reflect the complexity of the 'other' profession's role, nor it could be argued, particularly advance the student's own professional understandings. The use of the Framework allows students to access these valuable opportunities but with a purpose of achieving incrementally more challenging interprofessional learning outcomes, thus raising the student's level of achievement, rather than regressing it.

- ## The Capability Framework brings the patient to the foreground

  The NHS Improvement Plan (DH, 2004) underlines the need for the National Health Service to be 'patient driven'. A focus on interprofessional capability through use of the Framework not only emphasises the centrality of the patient for students' learning and assessment, but also reflects how interprofessional working occurs when services are structured around the patient. Students' attention being drawn through the Framework to observing the multidisciplinary team at work *for* the patient. Such attention to the needs of the patient also facilitates greater understanding of the roles and changing roles of different disciplines, and how that impacts upon care provision.

- **The complexity of the Framework**

  Despite a general agreement of the capabilities and learning outcomes contained in the Framework being appropriate and reflecting the realities of interprofessional working, some practitioners commented on certain statements being overly complex. The Interprofessional Capability Framework was developed from the QAA benchmarks, thus indicating the level of practice that students emerging as qualified practitioners should attain and the learning levels within the Framework attempt to provide a graduated development. However, this issue highlights the tensions concerning the expectations of newly qualified practitioners with respect to skill level, and the level of responsibility, seen as appropriate for them to have been given as students, in order to learn and be prepared for qualified roles. In turn, this may indicate the need for staff and service development, in order for students to be appropriately supported as student practitioners.

Key points arising from students' self-assessment of their interprofessional capability are shown in Box 4.6:

Box 4.6 Student Self-Assessment

Students were able to recognise and assess their interprofessional learning whilst in practice, and grade their level of achievement against the learning outcomes contained in the Framework.

Students were often able to apply and transfer or integrate the theoretical context of interprofessional learning which had been learned within the classroom to the practice based learning experience. This linking of theory to practice enabled students to progress their learning, and achieve higher levels of capability.

> **Box 4.6 (Continued)**
>
> Students were able to discriminate between the levels of achievement. Interestingly, where students placed themselves on the Framework was related not to their seniority in terms of years of study, or related to their profession, but depended on the length of experience they had accrued in practice.

Evaluation of the Capability Framework's utility as an assessment focus revealed the following:

- Practitioners found the Framework helpful and, to a large extent, user-friendly. They believed it could have a practical application in assessing student interprofessional learning in practice areas, although issues around language and terminology could present some barriers and may need to be addressed.
- The Framework provoked consideration of the perspective of the professional background of the student, and practitioners felt that they needed to have confidence in their knowledge and understanding of the roles of the interprofessional team, in order to assess students from another profession.
- The practitioners considered that the Framework reflected the dimension of interprofessional working, and indicated that it also validated their own interprofessional practice.
- The use of a tool that addresses the capabilities of all professions to interprofessional working provides a focus for assessing students from another profession during an interprofessional mentoring encounter.
- The use of an interprofessional assessment tool common to all students was considered to have the potential to ensure equity for students and would motivate students to fuller engagement, when being provided with interprofessional learning opportunities.

Applying the Interprofessional Framework Within the Curriculum

The Interprofessional Learning Framework is offered to colleagues as a flexible tool, with which to guide students' development as collaborative workers. Various examples have been given to us of how it has been utilised with or without adaptation, across a number of settings and contexts in the UK and in other English-speaking countries, at both undergraduate and postgraduate levels. Within our own institution, it has also been used in diverse ways. The capabilities have previously been incorporated into the practice learning assessment documents of one profession where they were successfully assessed in tandem with the students' more profession-specific practice learning outcomes.

More recently, we have embedded the Framework capabilities and competencies into the core interprofessional learning curriculum. The interprofessional core curriculum is accessed by all health, social care and social work students and comprises six modules. Two modules are studied in each year of the student's course: Introduction to Interprofessional Practice; Using Knowledge and Evidence to Support Study and Practice; Developing Collaborative Practice; Using and Evaluating Evidence to Inform Practice; Capable Collaborative Working; and Generating and Evaluating Evidence for Practice.

These modules represent elements of common, shared and interprofessional learning. Box 4.7 identifies our definitions of these terms:

Box 4.7 Definitions of Common, Shared and Interprofessional Learning

Common learning indicates that students across our professional programmes follow the same modules but not together in multidisciplinary groups and not necessarily at the same time. This is represented in the Using Knowledge and Evidence to Support Study and Practice that students access in the first year of their course and the Generating and Evaluating Evidence for Practice module that students access in the final year of a three year course. All students access these modules but they are delivered and studied in uniprofessional groups.

Shared learning indicates that students from our professional programmes access common modules and study within these modules at the same time 'side by side' in multiprofessional groupings. This is represented in the Using and Evaluating Evidence to Inform Practice, where students access in mixed profession groups, with some uniprofessional tutorial support.

Interprofessional learning indicates that students access common modules at the same time, side by side with students from other professional programmes but with the express purpose of learning with, from and about each other in order to improve collaboration and the quality of care (Barr, 2002). This is represented in the Introduction to Interprofessional Practice; Developing Collaborative Practice and Capable Collaborative Working modules where students study in mixed professional groups.

All of these modules, whether common, shared or interprofessional, are designed to address the capabilities contained in the Framework. The Framework is introduced to students as a reflective learning journal at the beginning of their university career. They are asked to maintain this journal during the course of their total programme. Students are encouraged to draw upon all aspects of their learning: within the designated core interprofessional curriculum, their profession-specific learning and practice learning, to chart their development as collaborative workers against the capabilities contained in the Framework. The modules that are defined above as 'interprofessional' carry assessment components where students are expected to make an assessment of their emerging interprofessional capability and plan future learning and development. In the final year of the students' course, they are asked to project this development into their first year of qualified practice.

Supporting the Development of Interprofessional Capability

Pedagogical approach

Recent work conducted with lecturers, involved in the delivery of the interprofessional core curriculum, has resulted in an articulation of a pedagogical approach to support the development of interprofessional capability. The data collected were reflective of the ongoing development of learning and teaching strategies. This included the lecturers' engagement with e learning supported by the Centre for Interprofessional e learning, a collaborative Centre for Excellence in Teaching and Learning between Coventry University and Sheffield Hallam University. The approaches identified by the lecturers, as informing how they design learning, teaching and assessment strategies to support the development of interprofessional capability, were as follows:

- *The employment of constructivist learning approaches – including a blended learning approach using adult learning theories, active learning and small group strategies*

  Our IPE programme is delivered via blended learning, using the Blackboard Virtual Learning Environment (VLE) for online and other e learning strategies, and also using direct tutor-facilitated sessions with smaller groups of students. The strategies employed do address informational issues regarding underpinning concepts; these are most often delivered via e lectures and other online learning approaches. However, with increasing emphasis, as students progress through the years of their professional courses, the programme concentrates on encouraging them to share their personal knowledge bases with each other, thus generating new (interprofessional) knowledge between them (i.e. learning with, from and about each other).

- *Placing the patient/client/service user/carer at the centre of the learning*

  The constructive approaches described above take place in a context of service user centredness. The students are offered opportunities to work together on scenarios and stories that involve practice based issues and together they complete tasks that require collaboration. The lecturers report the active involvement of service users in the planning and development of learning materials.

- *Focusing on practice*

  Learning materials and assessment activities within the interprofessional programme are focused on practice based issues. In common with other universities engaged in providing IPE, we experience logistical problems of ensuring students can be offered opportunities to learn with, from and about each other. These issues are addressed through the use of online learning sets, within which students can continue to engage in collaborative tasks, even when distributed across the UK undertaking placement learning.

- *Providing 'authentic' learning opportunities*

  In keeping with the notion of service user/carer centredness, the lecturers ensure that the learning materials and tasks used with students can be experienced as 'real' to their practice. Our work with service users and other experts to create and/or validate these materials is a strong component of our educational practice.

- *Professionally relevant*

  The lecturers recognise that students find it difficult to engage with learning materials that do not appear to be immediately relevant to their profession. These issues are mediated through providing scenarios and stories that students can recognise as being associated with their profession.

These factors are seen by the lecturers as important to consider when planning teaching to facilitate the development of interprofessional capability. They reported e learning as helpful in overcoming some of the reported barriers to interprofessional learning (Thistlethwaite and Nisbet, 2007). Online learning is an obvious solution to the notorious logistical difficulties of getting very large numbers of students, from varied courses together to learn with, from and about each other (Barr, 2002). However, the lecturers report that a blended approach that offers students the opportunity to learn online, for example accessing e-lectures, but also come together in actuality, is powerful. E-materials delivered in a classroom and/or online offer the opportunity to present students with authentic, practice-focused, patient/service user–centred situations that students could actively engage with together.

Facilitation to promote interprofessional capability

Difficulties for teaching staff, in both campus and practice contexts, engaged in interprofessional teaching have been reported (Pearson *et al.*, 2007), and are probably more prevalent than the literature suggests. Pearson *et al.* (2007:27) report some of these difficulties being concerned with anxieties around 'having to know all the answers'. This has also been our experience, when discussing IPE in staff development sessions. Individuals new to interprofessional teaching frequently express concerns around not knowing about the substantive content of students' disciplines other than their own. We attempt to address some of these anxieties by encouraging teachers, contributing to our programme, to adopt a model of interprofessional facilitation that has been developed through the previous project that incorporates notions of interprofessional capability (Marshall and Gordon, 2004). The model was developed within the context of practice based learning, but we consider it easily translates to campus teaching.

The work involved a form of concept analysis loosely based on the work of Walker and Avant (1988) and Chinn and Jacobs (1987). Walker and Avant discuss three ways of defining the attributes of a concept – analysis (describing and explicating), synthesis (deriving new concepts) and translating concepts across disciplines (concept derivation). At the outset of the work, it seemed clear from our knowledge of practice that support of learners (pre- and post-qualified) was taking place across the professions in practice settings, indicating that the notion of synthesis might then be somewhat stretched. Also, due to the paucity of literature that defines the concept of interprofessional facilitation, examining the steps of conceptualisation, suggested by all the authors, seemed to indicate that analysis of existing definitions would be problematic; however, translating across disciplines was of obvious importance. Following Walker and Avant (1988) and Chinn and Jacobs (1987), the aim was to develop a model case whilst also following advice from Rodgers (2000), to produce the example from empirical work. This was undertaken by conducting qualitative interviews with students, and practitioners who support students of their own and other professions.

In summary, a model case (Figure 4.1) was developed by formulating a working definition of interprofessional facilitation (or mentorship), and articulating the processes involved. This model identifies that the facilitation task in interprofessional learning is concerned with the promotion of collaborative skills and the knowledge and attitudes that underpin these, and that this knowledge is common to all professions and so available to all academics engaged in the programme, no matter

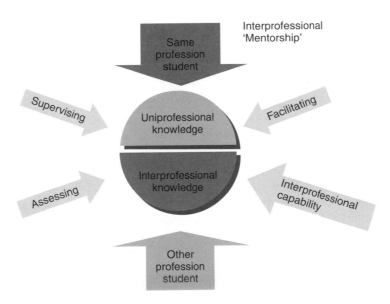

Figure 4.1 A model of Interprofessional Mentorship
Source: Gordon and Marshall (2005) CUILU

their professional background, and no matter that the students they are teaching are not of their profession.

The model contends that when working with students from both the same profession and other professions, a central consideration is the type of knowledge that the student and teacher are engaging with, in order to facilitate learning. In interprofessional teaching, the facilitator is able to draw on two aspects of knowledge: that which is specific to their own profession, and that which is more generic and relevant to all professions – interprofessional knowledge. For example, when teaching a student from his/her own profession, the facilitator draws on uniprofessional knowledge for profession-specific teaching, but may also draw on interprofessional knowledge to aid that student's more general professional development and gaining of interprofessional capability.

However, when teaching a student of another profession, the facilitator draws mainly on interprofessional knowledge to help the student gain skills and attributes, necessary for interprofessional capability. In tandem with this, the mentor may draw on his/her uniprofessional knowledge to teach this student aspects of the mentor's own profession useful to the student's learning, about holistic aspects of caring for patients/service users. This model can be extended to include notions of constructivist approaches in more autonomous, student-directed interprofessional learning, where students learn with, from and about each other by not only sharing common 'interprofessional' knowledge, but also exchanging their uniprofessional perspectives to generate new insights into their knowledge repertoires.

Conclusion

The Interprofessional Capability Framework was devised to provide guidance to teachers and students about learning which needs to occur in order to develop the collaborative workers required for contemporary health, social work and social care services. We intended that our colleagues would use it flexibly and according to the needs of their situation. We have used the capabilities and their building competencies in different ways and have more recently embedded it into the curriculum as a reflective tool, with the interprofessional programme being designed around the knowledge, skills and attitudes contained within it. Its use is still emerging and requires robust evaluation; however, we recognise that practice and our knowledge bases are constantly evolving and that this may impact on its utility and relevance. The Framework was developed through grounded theory analytic processes (Glaser and Strauss, 1967; Charmaz, 1995). These strategies allow us to revisit the Framework in the light of new data, for example, revisions of the QAA benchmarks and rising priorities in policy that may affect the conceptualisation of domains and the nature of the capabilities and competencies contained within it.

Notes

1. The Combined Universities Interprofessional Learning Unit – a collaborative initiative between Sheffield Hallam University and Sheffield University funded by the Department of Health. Permission granted by the universities for material within the chapter.
2. see www.cipel.ac.uk

References

Barr, H. (2002). *Interprofessional Education: Today, Yesterday and Tomorrow*. London: LTSN – Centre for Health Sciences and Practice.

Charmaz, K. (1995). Grounded theory. In J.A. Smith, R. Harre and L.V. Langenhove (eds) *Rethinking Methods in Psychology*. London: Sage, Chapter 3, pp. 27–49.

Chinn, K.R. and M.K. Jacobs. (1987). *Theory and Nursing: A Systematic Approach*. St Louis: Mosby.

DH. (1997). *Better Services for Vulnerable People*. London: Department of Health, The Stationery Office.

DH. (1999). *National Service Frameworks for Mental Health: Modern Standards and Service Models*. London: Department of Health, The Stationery Office.

DH. (2000). *The NHS Plan*. London: Department of Health, The Stationery Office.

DH. (2001). *Valuing People a New Strategy for Learning Disability for the 21st Century a White Paper*. London: Department of Health, The Stationery Office.

DH. (2002). *The Expert Patient: A New Approach to Cronic Disease Management for the 21st Century*. London: Department of Health, The Stationery Office.

DH. (2004). *The NHS Improvement Plan: Putting People at the Heart of Public*. London: Department of Health, The Stationery Office.

Fraser, S. and T. Greenhalgh (2001). Coping with complexity: Educating for capability. *British Medical Journal* 323 (7316), 799–803.

Freeth, D., M. Hammick, I. Koppel, S. Reeves and H. Barr. (2002). *A Critical Review of Evaluations of Interprofessional Education*. Working Paper. Higher Education Academy, Health Sciences and Practice Network, London, UK.

Glaser, B.G. and A. Strauss. (1967). *The Discovery of Grounded Theory*. New York: Aldine Publishing Company.

Gordon, F., C. Walsh, M. Marshall, F. Wilson and T. Hunt. (2004). Developing interprofessional capability in students of health and social care – the role of practice-based learning. *Journal of Integrated Care* 12 (4), 12–18.

Gordon, F., C. Walsh, M. Marshall, F. Wilson and T. Hunt. (2006). *The Combined Universities Interprofessional Learning Unit: Final Report*. Sheffield Hallam University and University of Sheffield. ISBN 184 387 2188.

Gordon, F. and C. Walsh. (2005). A framework for interprofessional capability: Developing students of health and social care as collaborative workers. *Journal of Integrated Care* 13 (3), 26–33.

Gordon F. and K. Ward. (2005). Making it real: Interprofessional teaching strategies in practice. *Journal of Integrated Care* 13 (5), 42–47.

Hagar, P. and A. Gonezi. (1996). What is competence? *Medical Teacher* 18 (1), 15–18.

Hall, P. and L. Weaver. (2001). Interdisciplinary education and teamwork: A long and winding road. *Medical Education* 35 (9), 867–875.

Heron G. and R. Murray. (2004). The place of writing in social work: Bridging the theory-practice divide. *Journal of Social Work* 4 (2), 199–214.

Kennedy, I. (2001). *The Bristol Royal Infirmary Inquiry*. CM5207 (1). London: HMSO.

Knowles, M.S. (1990). *The Adult Learner: A Neglected Species* (4th Edition). Houston: Gulf Publishing Company.

Laming, Lord. (2003). *The Victoria Climbié Inquiry*. Norwich: HMSO.

Marshall, M. and F. Gordon. (2004). Interprofessional mentorship: Taking on the challenge. *Journal of Integrated Care* 13 (2), 38–43.

McCray, J. (2003). Leading interprofessional practice: A conceptual framework to support practitioners in the field of learning disability. *Journal of Nursing Management* 11 (6), 387–395.

Pearson, P., C. Dickinson, A. Steven and P. Dawson. (2007). Towards a common goal: Developing practice based interprofessional education in North East England. In Barr, H. (ed.) *Piloting Interprofessional Education: Four English Case Studies*. London: The Higher Education Academy.

QAA. (2000). *Social Policy and Administration and Social Work: Subject Benchmarking Statements*. Bristol: Quality Assurance Agency for Higher Education.

QAA. (2001). *Benchmarking Academic and Practitioner Standards in Health Care Subjects*. Bristol: Quality Assurance Agency for Higher Education.

QAA. (2002). *Medicine: Subject Benchmarking Statements*. Bristol: Quality Assurance Agency for Higher Education.

Rodgers, B.L. (2000). Concept analysis: An evolutionary view. In B.L. Rodgers and K.A. Knaft (eds) *Concept Development in Nursing: Foundations Techniques and Applications*. Philidelphia: Saunders, pp. 77–102.

Rushmer, R. (2005). Blurred boundaries damage interprofessional working. *Nurse Researcher* 12 (3), 74–84.

SCMH. (2001). *The Capable Practitioner*. London: The Sainsbury Centre for Mental Health.

Thistlethwaite, J. and G. Nisbet. (2007). Interprofessional education: What's the point and where we're at. *The Clinical Teacher* 4 (2), 67–72.

Walker, K. and K. Avant. (1988). *Strategies for Theory Construction in Nursing*. London: Appleton and Lang.

Walsh, C., F. Gordon, M. Marshall, F. Wilson and T. Hunt. (2005). Interprofessional Capability: A developing framework for interprofessional education. *Nurse Education in Practice* 5 (4), 230–237.

Wilson, T. and T. Holt. (2001). Complexity and clinical care. *British Medical Journal* 323, 685–688.

Part II
Interprofessional Education Approaches

This part of the book is made up of two chapters. In Chapters 5 and 6 the editors describe their own experiences of implementing both face-to-face and e-based interprofessional education (IPE). Both chapters relate to models of IPE, focusing on accounts both of the development and implementation of face-to-face methods of IPE as well as online e learning approaches.

It could be argued that IPE learning lends itself, even begs itself to be delivered face to face and preferably in practice, but although there are advantages to this method of delivery, there are also challenges and disadvantages to this not only in the number of students, but also the different placement learning outcomes across professional groups. Online learning provides a different method which can be less intrusive on uni-professional curricula and may be seen to interfere less with timetabling issues, but it must be remembered that it does not afford the face-to-face and applied learning of IPE in practice. Each has its own strengths and weaknesses, each its own challenges. This part of the book uses the editors' experiences of the two models extensively as examples – both methods are developmental and therefore aspects within them have changed over time and continue to evolve in response to student and facilitator feedback and experiences. However, they do provide the reader with a step-by-step guide to two methods of delivery of IPE which do not involve a complete curriculum overhaul. At the end of Chapter 5 there are many examples of other UK and international models of IPE in practice which the reader may find useful.

5

A Practice Model of Interprofessional Education

Ann Jackson and Patricia Bluteau

Introduction

There are numerous models, programmes and initiatives of interprofessional education (IPE) available in the literature (Anderson *et al.*, 2006; Lindqvist *et al.*, 2005; Reeves and Freeth, 2002); some of these models involve whole curricula change (O'Halloran *et al.*, 2006), whilst others are interwoven throughout uniprofessional programmes (Bluteau and Jackson 2005; Lennox and Anderson 2007).

Freeth *et al.* (2001) suggest that 'Practice based interprofessional learning is more effective than a theory based intervention in generating positive behaviour and organisational/patient outcomes.' For us, there is little doubt that creating interprofessional activities in practice is received and evaluated extremely positively by both students and professional staff. We think that this is because of its applied nature.

The IPE activity, we are going to describe, is one which we piloted five years ago, and which now runs each year. It is sustainable, low cost and low on resources. It has been evaluated positively every year, by both participating students and qualified professionals alike. This activity allows students, working as a team, to take responsibility for the care of two patients for a week, whilst providing them with the support of and access to experienced professionals based on the ward. Through this activity we have observed the development of a student team (all members were previously unknown to each other), showing signs of not only cooperative working but more importantly collaborative working (see Chapter 10).

We firmly believe that if IPE activities are to become part of a placement experience, they need to be efficient in terms of human

---

Box 5.1 Five Key Elements Crucial to Successful Collaborative Working (D'Eon 2005)

- Positive interdependence
- Face-to-face promotive interaction
- Individual accountability
- Interpersonal and small group skills
- Group processing

---

resources, time and cost, whilst at the same time providing a positive learning opportunity for students, where students can learn with, from and about each other without detracting or interfering with each student's placement learning outcomes.

This model of IPE uses key educational principles and practices as suggested by D'Eon (2005) as a blueprint for interprofessional learning (Box 5.1).

Initial Contacts

Senior managers and heads of departments across participating universities and trusts were approached to obtain permission for their students/staff to be involved within the pilot. The universities provided the names, numbers and year of training of potential students. The heads of departments within the trusts identified key staff (mentors/practice tutors) that had students on placement.

A series of meetings were undertaken at each of the sites, involving all the front-line individuals and the overall aim of the week long pilot was identified. The following topics (Box 5.2) were identified as requiring consideration between the professionals:

Box 5.2 Topics for Consideration

- Number, discipline, make up of students;
- Number, medical condition and stage of recovery of the patients;
- Structure of the week;
- Aim and learning outcomes of the week;

- Establishing a balance between uniprofessional and interprofessional learning;
- Developing the role of the 'experts';
- Setting the aim of the week within a service setting;
- Establishing a role for the students – balancing interprofessional and uniprofessional working;
- Developing the role of facilitators.

The week long activity was designed in collaboration with mentors and practice educators who were already responsible for their own professional students, when they were out on placement. The activity was shaped to include the normal make up and number of students who worked on each ward. As all wards worked in multidisciplinary teams, the idea of a student led multidisciplinary team seemed a natural choice of activity.

The main areas of concern for staff hinged on whether participating in this week long activity would be met with resistance, and whether there would be problems meeting the needs of all the students and would therefore have little chance of sustainability in the future. The clinical staff, whose students were participating in the IPL week discussed these areas of concern as a group. The ward manager who was extremely keen to run the week and who became the placement champion offered to act as a joint facilitator for the student group, provided that the practice educator, allocated to the rehabilitation unit, would act as the other facilitator. By so doing, all mentors were able to take on the role of 'experts' for the week, whilst the facilitators supported the student group on a daily basis. The facilitators agreed that they would be available for 30 minutes every day to support interprofessional learning and teamworking and to ensure that students had time to raise any problems or seek advice.

Although all students, irrespective of professional background, were able to access any of the 'experts' it became apparent that, as on any normal placement, experts were more likely to be used by their own student for uniprofessional advice. This was an important part of the week, by providing each student with expert knowledge, support was easily accessible on a daily basis, if needed. In this way, if a student was unsure of their own role in the care of the patients they were able to 'check' before raising it within the student group. In reality, students used their experts, prior to the multidisciplinary team meeting to ensure that their management plans and goals for each patient were correct.

Students

Every mentor on the participating wards was included; this meant that their students were involved in the team. Once the week had been identified by the mentors, they individually contacted their students to discuss whether the students were happy to participate in the week. Student guides had been developed and given to each student (Appendix 1). The learning outcomes for the week were included in the student guide (Box 5.3).

Whilst students may be anxious about participating, no one has refused yet. It is made very clear to them that this is a voluntary activity and that non-participation will not affect their placement grades.

In the student guide there are some activities, which students are encouraged to complete and bring with them on the first day. One of these activities asks students to self-report, using a likert scale, on their knowledge of other professional roles, the function of a multidisciplinary team and any thoughts they have on the impact of teamworking on patient care (Appendix 2). They are also asked to consider/record their own ideas of the roles and responsibilities of a list of health and social care professionals who are often involved in rehabilitation/stroke units. Each year medical, nursing and physiotherapy students participate, with an occupational therapy/pharmacy and/or speech and language therapy student if any are out on placement.

Box 5.3 Aim and Learning Outcomes of Interprofessional Learning Week

- Aim
- To participate in a multiprofessional group to explore the care of an allocated patient(s).
- Learning Outcomes
- By the end of the week, students will be able to
- Recognise the importance of teamworking to deliver effective patient care
- Begin to compare and contrast the different skills of team members
- Appreciate the importance of placing the patient, and the patient's views at the centre of teamworking
- Actively engage in reviewing the case of an individual patient(s) with members of their own/other profession(s)
- Discuss their patient(s) at a student led multidisciplinary team meeting

Plan of the Week

At the beginning of the week, the students and facilitators meet. Each 'expert' has an allocated 10 minute slot to briefly describe their role on the ward. Each student has a workbook, outlining the learning outcomes and plan of the week.

After coffee, the student teams are told the names of the two patients they will be responsible for during the week. (The patients are chosen by the 'experts' and are consented by the ward manager.) At the end of the week the student team present the care, treatment and management plan of their patients at a student multidisciplinary team meeting.

Students are charged with working as a team, planning the daily care and developing a management plan with appropriate goals for each patient. They are also advised not to limit themselves to their own professions, but to assess each patient and if they feel, in their clinical opinion, they wish to refer their patient, then they are encouraged to make contact with that specific profession and discuss their referral. In this way the student group is able to work together to provide person-centred care. Often the students will identify several professions they wish to meet with regarding possible involvement in the patient's care, for example psychologists, discharge coordinators and even support groups who they feel their patients might benefit from now or in the future. The students agree between themselves who will meet with each profession; usually this meeting involves at least two students. After the meeting they will discuss as a group the outcome of each meeting.

Students are left to decide how to plan their week – they know that the emphasis is on cooperative teamworking; they know that they have two patients to care for; they know that at the end of the week they will be expected to present the two patients at a student led multidisciplinary team, in front of their mentors (Experts). How they achieve this is left for them to decide. This lack of structure acts as an ice breaker; students are forced to discuss how they are going to achieve this over a one-week period.

Choosing Your Site(s)

Initially, several wards may be keen to participate – we have found that this usually takes the shape of at least one interested and enthusiastic professional – for example on one ward this turned out to be the consultant, on another it was the physiotherapist and on two others it was the ward managers (both nurses). These key people become the champions on each ward, supported by the university lead. Being ward-based and knowing other members of the team, as well as working on a daily basis and over a period of time, help disseminate the idea of IPE in practice and preparations can begin in earnest once a champion has come forward. Using the MDT as the IPE activity means that theoretically it can be used in any setting where MDTs are a routine part of patient care/ward activity and where students are placed.

Our Experience

Initially, we had four wards from a large acute teaching hospital and one ward from a rehabilitation community hospital. All of the wards had similar numbers of students – although there tended to be more nursing students on wards based in the acute hospital.

Physiotherapists, nurses and medics tended to be the most accessible with occupational therapists and speech and language therapists being the least. Dietetic students were never available, as their four year course did not involve any placements.

The challenges to implementing a week long activity continued despite the support and engagement of champions on each ward. This took many different shapes and has been reported more fully in the literature (Jackson and Bluteau 2007; Barker *et al.*, 2005; Gilbert 2005), and in Chapter 10. Briefly, there were difficulties in engaging some of the other members of the team which not only impacted on the development of the activity, but also highlighted weaknesses between members of the MDT team. For example, one of the professionals booked study leave one week before the IP week commenced, despite the teams' joint decision on that week, having been made months before. These external stresses impacted heavily on team dynamics and suggested to us that where team members were suddenly unable to participate (despite months of preparation), such teams had members who worked as a cooperative team rather than as a collaborative team. To an outsider, these wards were functioning as MDT teams, but we feel that this was at the level of cooperative working. We base this on the following definition by Roschelle and Teasley (1995), who suggest that the difference between cooperative working and collaboration is '*Cooperative work may be where the task is divided into bits so each person has responsibility for one portion – collaboration is the motivational engagement of participants in a coordinated effort to solve the problem.'*

Teams working cooperatively have some members who are not as willing to participate in activities which involve students other than their own professional group, whether this reflects a lack of confidence is not clear. Whatever the reason, these teams do not succeed in managing students during the IP week activity. Perhaps though, the most fascinating aspect of this for us was that one student who had not been supported by her mentor was interviewed after the activity. The lack of support and the distancing of just this one mentor who failed to engage had a huge impact on this student. Interestingly, the other students had tried to overcome these difficulties, during the week, by attempting to engage with the student, but had realised that this was placing the student in a difficult position, in relation to her own professional team and personal mentor, so they had reluctantly not persevered. Below are some of the comments from the unsupported student.

> *I mean they let my mentor know, but that would be the practice educators. They sort of came on and told my mentor half way through the week, because the other staff seemed to be unaware of what we were doing. And sometimes . . . I don't think I spent that much time with the actual patients. I remember, sort of, half way through the week, I made a real effort to go and sit and talk with him. And then it was, sort of, some of the other staff were a bit – oh, why is she only, you know, talking to that one patient. So I think if everyone knew you were taking part, you wouldn't feel so bad about going off and talking to the one patient.*
>
> (Female Student Nurse K05)

> *'Cos at one stage, I said to my mentor, 'oh, I'm going to talk to the patient,' and she actually said to me, 'we're a bit short staffed today, if I have to call you away, you'll have to come and do something else.' Which I felt was a bit unfair, because we are supernumerary and . . . it was really a learning. . . . For everyone, even those taking part. I felt like we could learn a lot, by talking to the medics, the physios. Especially physios, 'cos even with the students, we don't do a lot together.*
>
> (Female Student Nurse K05)

All the other students were also interviewed individually following the week long activity. Each student (including the unsupported student) overwhelmingly supported the aim of the week and recommended that it should be repeated. Their only one stipulation was that to be successful then professional staff had to support and facilitate the activity. It seems that this type of activity is able to identify weak or debilitated multidisciplinary teams. Where functioning teams exist, as in the rehabilitation unit (Chapter 10), not only do students really benefit and develop in terms of knowledge and confidence but so do members of the existing team – in some cases this type of activity serves to increase the skills and confidence of both students and participating professionals – a win–win situation.

When choosing a site – especially if it is to act as a model for other sites – explore how the professional team works together, notice the off-duty activity, the daily conversations with each other, the institutional stressors and the impact on staff morale – how does this impact on the IP team – do they 'moan' together or uniprofessionally about daily demands.

The site that worked in our case was a ward where staff often met off duty, where daily conversation was not just about work, but also involved personal aspects of life. It was on a non-acute unit which meant that it was free from the stresses associated with main stream acute hospitals. We do believe that this IP week will work in an acute setting with a cooperative working team but the champions would need a higher level of support and staff preparation, for the activity would need to be spread over a long period of time.

Observations of the Week

The collaborative model explained in Chapter 10 provides in more detail changes observed during the week, between the students and participating professional staff. Students were given timetables which had a few specific commitments but a good deal of time which could be used to explore uniprofessional or interprofessional roles and responsibilities necessary for the care of their patients (Appendix 3). Students communicated from day one, and as they exchanged ideas and asked questions of each other (often to clarify uniprofessional jargon), their confidence began to develop, irrespective of their stage of training. They began to realise that they had something to offer to the group – be it in translating jargon or clarifying different aspects of the ward, their own professional routine, or aspects of their own training programme. The commonality of being a student helped reduce the vulnerability which had been felt initially by most of the student group with respect to what other students would expect of them. For example, medics were anxious that they did not know enough to participate and that other students would expect them to know 'medical' aspects of the disease – usually management of the disease – which they felt they had yet to cover. In reality, students were far more interested in learning the anatomy or mechanisms of the disease process, or what their course was like, and this the medical students did know. Student nurses were often anxious about their perceived lower level of educational attainment and how the pitch of learning might be difficult for them. In reality, student nurses had a much greater experience of working in practice and so had a greater understanding of pathways of care and usual input (not only of their own profession, but also of when patients might be referred to other professionals, and routine observations and tests which might be needed).

As the week progressed students spent more time together – going to breaks and lunches together, coming in early to accommodate each other's different working patterns. By the end of the week the group was relaxed with each other. The student led multidisciplinary team meeting allowed the students to showcase their findings and decisions in relation to the two patients; it also provided an opportunity for all mentors to come together and witness the whole student group effort. This seemed to help reinforce to the mentors the potential learning for all students, but especially their own – it was this trigger, along with the knowledge, that the week had not increased their own workload or impacted on their own student's learning, which generated enthusiasm for continuing the week long activity.

The Role of the 'Experts'

The importance of the mentors is crucial to the success of the week: they lead on the uniprofessional perspective, assist their own students in any areas where they are not sure of their own role and they give credibility to the activity as they are clinicians working within the practice setting. This means that they are aware of how the ward environment is organised and are able to guide students where needed. They also act as role models, in that not only are they experienced working within multidisciplinary teams, but as a team of professionals they are known to each other and have an existing good working relationship on which students can role model. They provide an understanding/working knowledge of their uniprofessional perspective to the student group on the first morning of the IP week. They also provide support and guidance to their own student as necessary and are available at two key points during the week:

- First morning of pilot week
- MDT

The mentors, along with the facilitators, play a key role in the week long activity. We found that they are able to empower, enable and develop the student team by positive engagement, support and role model. Through their actions students are able to develop both uniprofessionally and interprofessionally.

Facilitator Role

The facilitation role, similar to the experts role, is essential to implementing interprofessional learning in pre-registration education. Facilitation sessions should be timetabled throughout the week. Initially we allocated 60 minutes, on a daily basis, however these were reduced to 30 minutes when it became evident that the students did not need this amount of time. By year three, this had further reduced to times of 10–30 minutes and was not necessarily needed on a daily basis although the option for longer and more frequent contact was always available. The remit of the facilitator role is to guide the students and to ensure that as a group they are provided with the opportunity:

- to learn from, with and about each other;
- to understand and respect each other's roles in their patient(s) case;
- to work together as a team;
- to maintain, as a team, the focus of patient-centred care;
- to discuss each other's roles;
- to identify if and where their roles overlap in the care of their patient(s);
- to identify who will be responsible for the different aspects of care needed by their patient(s).

The facilitators create a safe learning environment which fosters mutual respect. This space gives students permission to explore their own and each other's roles, to challenge preconceptions and stereotypes, and to develop the MDT meeting in a new and creative format. During the week the role of the facilitators evolves in response to the students' needs. As the students gain confidence within their team, the role of the facilitators becomes less directive.

For the first few years we have used two facilitators. One facilitator helps the group to establish and adhere to ground rules for the week's work, usually by listening to the group's discussion, by asking questions and by creating a safe nurturing environment enabling the students to work together. We see this role as ensuring mutual respect and equal voices among the student team.

The other facilitator ensures that the group maintains its focus on the delivery of patient-centred and individualised care by assistance, direction, suggestion and intervention where necessary.

Both facilitators guide the group by initiating and monitoring the activities of the student team. They are also key to ensuring that each team member has a role, that students consider their role holistically and aid the development of collaboration and teamworking.

In between facilitation sessions, students work on the ward looking after their patients, working at times either as an interprofessional team or within their uniprofessional role.

The facilitators are able to suggest areas for further exploration, identify where to access further information or how to access relevant professionals.

They play a key role in challenging any student assumptions, which may have become apparent especially in relation to different professional roles and/or stereotypes, and they are present at the student led multidisciplinary meeting. Once the IP activity becomes established, it is possible to use one facilitator; however, for the first few weeks it is better to have two facilitators who are able to support each other, as well as divide the workload.

Two Tips for Effective Facilitation

1. One year (fortuitously), we accidentally had two facilitators who were able to contribute different skills to the facilitation process due to their differing clinical backgrounds. This accidental combination of skills proved to be beneficial to the facilitating role and is worthwhile considering when recruiting to this role.

(we had) . . . two very different backgrounds, Chris was well placed being the manager on the ward where it took place because she knew very much about the systems, routine, specifics and clinical issues and my background being in mental health perhaps lent itself a bit more to the overall facilitation.

(Male Facilitator 1)

It was really good to have Andre, to bounce ideas off one another and because he comes from a different clinical background. Also he was not based here and was more objective. He was also used to dealing with students as a facilitator.

(Female Facilitator 2)

2. Plan ahead so that protected time is available to ensure that service demands do not encroach on student sessions.

I wasn't supernumerary for that week . . . so I ensured that there was enough trained staff about . . . and we planned it for after lunch which made it (facilitator meeting) as though there was a natural break in what I was doing anyhow so we went for lunch and then straight afterwards it was in to the meeting.

(Female Facilitator 2)

The role of the facilitator is key to the success of interprofessional learning and working as a team. Good facilitation provides an environment which ensures students have an equal voice and respect for one another, irrespective of the stage of their training. If facilitators are not skilled in working with diverse groups, it is crucial to provide training which should include the development of skills in working with interprofessional groups. In particular the training should focus on developing group cohesion, building trust and mutual respect, developing authority and the ability to challenge and developing new perspectives, all of which was valued by the students.

Evaluation

Evaluating any new activity is essential, not only to refine and develop it for future years but also to measure whether the learning outcomes have been achieved. There is still very little evidence to support the belief that IPE improves collaboration and teamworking and so patient care. IPE is difficult to measure given that many of the changes relate to changing personal beliefs and attitudes. Chapters 7–9 provide some tools for evaluating IPE activities.

We have collected data pre- and post-IP week using a small simple questionnaire, followed up with 1:1 taped interviews aimed at capturing students' and experts' views in depth. The pre- and post-questionnaire (Appendix 2) consisted of six statements and asked students to agree or disagree with each statement using a likert scale (score 1 represented a poor understanding, 5 excellent understanding). At the end of the week, students were given another form with the same statements. These two forms were used to highlight any changes in student perception. Table 5.1 outlines the changes in perceived knowledge between the matched pre- and post-intervention questionnaires. Whilst it is recognised that this is a very small sample ($n = 10$) these findings were supported by qualitative data from the students, experts and facilitators.

Table 5.1 Self-Recorded Changes in Perceived Knowledge of Students pre- and Post-IP Activity

Statements (1 = poor understanding, 5 = excellent understanding)	Median likert score pre-MDT week	Median likert score post-MDT week	Significance (Mann Whitney)
My understanding of the roles of other health and social care professionals	3	4	0.002*
My understanding of my own profession's contribution in a team	4	4	NS
My understanding of the role of multidisciplinary meetings in the role of patient care	3	4.5	0.006
My understanding of the impact of interprofessional working on patient/client care	3	4	0.008
My understanding of the implications of 'key workers' in patient/client care	3	4	0.009
My understanding of how multidisciplinary working will impact on my postgraduate development	3	4	NS

* Statistically significant.

All 'experts' were also sent postal questionnaires and a sample was interviewed to explore their experiences in greater detail.

Students had valued participating in the student led MDT, of having the opportunity to work within an MDT and gain first-hand experience and insight into teamworking:

> *It was quite daunting, in a way, because I don't think any of us expected such a big audience. So I think…but apart from that, it was…it was good and I did get the feeling that everybody – everybody cared about the patients and everybody wanted to give their input. And I think the way we did it…obviously there were some technical hitches, but I think it did work quite well. Which was pleasing 'cos we had tried to break everything down and change it from the one we saw on the Monday, to try and improve it. I think some of that came through.*
>
> *(Female Student Medic E07)*

> *I said 'Is this correct? I feel that this is important and feel I am going to say this at the MDT?' and she (Expert) said 'Yeah, yeah you have got it to a tee, you have realised, you have discovered what the nurses role is and how extended the role has to be um'…and continue looking out for educating the patient being their advocate, umm…providing care for them, you know, it all slotted into place, you know.*
>
> *(Male Student Nurse L05 R)*

> *I mean the overall week, I think the idea to it, the basis was really good. And it should be repeated. 'Cos we always get told about the multidisciplinary teams, but while we're in practice it's really difficult to get involved with other people. 'cos, especially at the practice, 'cos you're so busy focusing on what you need to do, you kind of forget the other areas. So it's good in making students think about the other areas, they sort of relate to it.*
>
> *(Female Student Nurse K05 A)*

> *So it actually gave me a chance, to actually step back work with them and actually do a MDT for myself rather than just observing an MDT. It was a lot easier to take the role of professions and just sort of get stuck in rather than observing and sort of wondering what to say…No, I really enjoyed it and I actually found it very beneficial to take the time out…*
>
> *(Female newly qualified Physio PQ105)*

> *Because I was given my task to do, I felt more part of the team. Because it was a new environment I was bit unsure of what I had got to do 'Where's*

this?', 'Where's that?' but because the objectives were clear, everyone else knew that, that was our patient and we were supposed to care for that patient and tasks were left for us to do, instead of other members of the team coming across a problem and doing it, you know, it was nice to, you know, 'Mrs W, she's got this problem, you need to do this' . . . and it was nice from the fact, that I got more involved with the treatment and the care of them . . . and given my input as well.

(*Male Student Nurse L05 R*)

The students felt that they had learned about each other's roles and responsibilities and other team members not represented by students, such as discharge coordinators, psychologists, pharmacists, through discussion, information sharing and interviewing.

I remember one day, especially, it was quite – it's quite surprising to find out how similar the assessments that physios do on patients are to the ones that the medics do. And we weren't really aware of that and it's cross over, so it really brought all that home. All the . . . how things interlink and how the assessments are similar.

(*Female Student Medic E07*)

I learnt a lot from working with the nurses, I learnt a fair bit from working with the physio's. Generally I think, up till now we have been doing a morning with the physiotherapist or an afternoon with the district nurse and so having the time to spend a week working in close proximity with them, helping them with some of their tasks, getting their advice on what we were doing, I think that was really the key point that helped us learn.

(*Male Student Medic H05*)

I felt like a staff nurse, I didn't feel like a student. I had to think for myself, the support was there, if it was needed but it was nice to have this 'she is your patient, you look after her, you need to care for her and if you need you plan the care for her, you have to do it yourselves' and so if we came across a problem we had to communicate, we had to work them out together . . .

(*Male Student Nurse L05 R*)

because it was really interesting to see what the others really do and not what you think they do and to have that idea that we all are all coming with the same angle that we should be . . .

(*Female Student Nurse N05 R*)

> *talking to the pharmacy student on the Wednesday helped to bring it together a bit because she was talking about the drugs she was on, and none of us really knew how that was actually affecting her* (the patient). *So that was quite nice to bring that side of things into it. I wouldn't normally think of how medication might affect, but I should think it could be her medication and actually, I have had a few more patients since then, and I have thought actually, it may be their medication that's making her this way and that is why she is not responding...*
>
> (*Female newly qualified Physio PQ105*)

> *My other bit I think now I know it's more important to let other people know like, other people on the team know what you're doing as a nurse, whereas before I thought you just kept it amongst the nurses. Now I know it's important to let other people know cause it may be relevant. I might not think its relevant but it may to be to the other people on my disciplinary team.*
>
> (*Female Student Nurse E06*)

> *But then I can't really say...cos I know a first year student on the ward went to the presentation. She said, that was really good. She said, it's really good to see how it all came together and you got a really good picture about what our patient was. She said, you know, she could really see how much work we'd put into it.*
>
> (*Female Student Nurse K05A*)

Expert Role – From the Student and Expert Perspective

Students felt that the expert role was beneficial and found it useful in terms of support, advice and guidance especially when they were unclear of their own role.

> *when Chris introduced it 'This is the nurses role, this is what nurses do' and she broke it all down into bullet points 'This is the typical experts role...advocates' um can't remember all of it now but it all slotted into place there was a lot of templates that the nurse had to give. We certainly had to be care providers, we certainly had to be their advocate, reflecting on what every health professionals input, what ever they were giving her, for example she was quite low and depressed...having to comfort her and make her feel more positive about herself, making her look forward and not backwards um it was...it made me think...I think, at the beginning I was*

looking at the clinical side, I wasn't looking at the other side of things ... so it widened my horizons anyway, definitely and at the end it all clicked into place when I fed back to.

(*Male Student Nurse L05R*)

Well I think it gave them someone to go back to and someone to role model from because at the end of the day you have if you are saying right I am an OT student you have got to have a qualified OT and expert who says 'That's how the jobs done ... that's how you do it' ... you might have ideas about 'Well I might not do it quite like that, I might change that' – and that's fine but you have to have someone you can go back and say 'Right why are we doing this? Is there any reason why we can't do it like this?' and I think that that is quite important to get some feedback from as well.

(*Female Expert Nurse C05R*)

I mean some of the experts, we only had some of them there but I actually found that sheet quite useful, to actually write down the points of what you thought were the points of each profession was and then to feed back at the end of the week. My impression was very different after the week, even once being qualified I had a totally different view ...

(*Female newly qualified Physio PQ105*)

I could ask different nurses, I think coming on a Friday I was a bit unsure about a couple of things so I asked 2 different nurses what their views were so obviously, it wasn't, she (nurse expert) *wasn't in all the time so.*

(*Female Student Nurse E06R*)

Medics were the least supported in terms of accessing a mentor because this mentor relationship is not as clearly defined in medicine as it is in most other professionals. Special arrangements were therefore put in place for the medics – this took the shape of either consultants (not the best as their presence on the ward is often limited and therefore makes it more difficult for students to access them if they need advice) or Foundation Year (FY) 2 doctors – unfortunately there were difficulties here as well, with not all FY2 doctors willing to provide support despite having agreed prior to the activity.

I think if you ask a medic to do that, well from my own point of view, it'd be hard for me to make sometime every day to make sure things were going alright. Because I'm out at clinics and things and not necessarily on site. . . . So it was good to have somebody who did pop by and make contact

*with me . . . it was good from my point of view to know that that was going
to happen and if there were problems, somebody would pick it up.*

(Female Expert Medic M05)

The best mentor for the medics was on the rehabilitation ward
where a staff registrar enthusiastically supported and made herself
accessible to the medics – whether this reflected her long-term attach-
ment to the ward, there were less calls on her time, or that she saw
the importance of the activity (this is supported by her comment)
is not clear but both medics and other students benefited from her
participation.

*she was here you know 9–5 Monday to Friday and she oversaw them enthu-
siastically and they were made very keen . . . she used to sit down and do a
mock MDT with them anyway so she was very much into that and trying to
sort of say you are 'part of a team' and not just a medic who makes decision
on their own and that you would be making some hard decisions . . . about
treatment you need to be aware it is as part of a team.*

(Female Expert Nurse C05R)

*I think that it is good that the medical students get exposure early on in
their careers to teach them the concept of a MDT because I know medical
school teaching traditionally focuses on you as the doctor working alone
and sorting things out and in the real world it doesn't always work like
that so I think that it is a brilliant concept.*

(Female Expert Medic 06)

Initially, the experts had been concerned about the amount of time
this activity would take. However, following the activity, all of the
participating experts agreed that the increase on the demand of their
time had been negligible and that whatever they had put in was
worthwhile.

*they are asking questions so what you are doing and you are also advis-
ing, talking, showing them where they can get more information as well so
that does take time but it is doing it along side your normal job so . . . but
I felt personally and I know Dr Smith felt that it was a positive experience . . . anything that you had to spend time on it was far outweighed by
what you got back from it . . .*

(Female Expert Nurse C05R)

No I mean ideally the students would be here anyway wouldn't they? And so we would be spending time with them any way it is just a slightly different way of doing it? but I don't think it took up any more time than it would have done . . .

(*Female Expert Physio R05*)

No, they didn't come to me once, Glynis did, because obviously we were talking through her patients anyway, as we would just in a normal placement, but I don't suppose we actually talked about that particular patient any more that her other ones um . . . but no the nurse never came near me, nor did the medical students. Whether they gleaned enough from Glynis, as the physio . . . but no, I was never approached once . . .

(*Female Expert Physio A05*)

The experts particularly liked the use of the student led MDT and recommended this as an interprofessional learning activity and remarked that it encouraged some students to suggest improvements which could be made to the current weekly MDT meetings.

They (students) felt from the MDT, the one person that was missing, who was important, was the patient.

(*Female Expert Nurse 05*)

And as I say, I was actually, really, very pleasantly surprised what a professional job they did in terms of their feedback at the end and their synopsis and preparing together something that worked. And the other thing, that was very interesting was the team that was on our ward, I think, their presentation was very evenly based across the disciplines.

(*Female Expert Medic M05*)

I thought it all culminated in the MDT for me, that putting into practice. You can talk about something can't you, you can stand there and present, but when you are actually doing it, and when you are actually discussing a real patient, and they didn't miss anything, so it just shows they actually thought about it, carried that over and they actually took on the roles and divvied up what we do in the MDT – who was discussing what and they also overlapped as well, which is also important because we need to start looking at overlapping our roles and that can be hard sometimes when we have your own professional boundaries . . . so that, perhaps this way of learning is a way of doing that.

(*Female Expert Nurse 05*)

attending the MDT that they did at the end of the week – um I think they did that really well um…and it was a good setting to do it here because we have a good MDT running here in the rehab hosp.

(Female OT Expert R05)

Whilst the students enjoyed the experience, the experts were not so sure they had enjoyed it as much as the students (Table 5.2). When this was explored in greater depth it seemed to be related to being a 'first' time experience, where no one was sure how it would work – new and untested territory. The fact that all of them wanted to use the activity again suggested that it had not put anyone off!

Um…bit chaotic but it was a pilot, and I think from that point of view you know, it was a bit [of a] chaotic exercise but fundamentally underneath it is a good idea.

(Female Expert Physio A05)

So I think particularly if you're recruiting people who haven't done that kind of thing, haven't got involvement in inter professional learning in any way, then I would say, be very careful about giving them a clear brief, how to do this and how to pitch this.

(Female Expert Medic M05)

Um I think it needs if it runs again it needs to be discussed more with physios and OT's I think it was discussed at a higher level and not fed back down to us until a few weeks before.

(Female Physio Expert R05)

The quantitative data collected from a simple evaluation form (Appendix 4) (Table 5.2) supported these comments with students

Table 5.2 Comparison of Evaluation Feedback from Students and Experts

Likert scores of 4 and 5 (4 – agree, 5 = strongly agree)	Students (%)	Experts (%)
Student led multidisciplinary team meeting is a good IPE activity	91	88.3
I would recommend the interprofessional activity	72.8	100
I enjoyed participating in the interprofessional activity	82	66.7

and experts agreeing on the use of the MDT meeting as an IP activity and the most agreeing or strongly agreeing that it was worth recommending.

Facilitator Role

Students endorsed the need for support that was not didactic and which allowed space to explore new ways of working, with the opportunity to create new ideas within a safe and secure environment.

The ongoing need for daily facilitation appeared to be influenced by the student's stage of training. Once the facilitators had enabled the student group to gel, the perceived need for prescribed facilitation by the senior students but not the junior changed. It is suggested that this occurred as the confidence of the student team increased.

> *'And it was nice as well 'cos it went a lot more in depth talking about the patients so we kinda had sort of ideas that we might need to bring up in the meeting.... I felt it was nice just to have them there even if it was just one question that I needed to ask...'.*
>
> *(Female Student Nurse 07)*

> *I think it is important to have some kind of facilitation (interviewer on a daily basis?).... I think that could be up to the group...*
>
> *(Female Student Physio 07)*

> *I think her role was really to bring us together at a set time when we could all sit down talk but she was sort of um ... perhaps throwing different ideas at us if we were coming up with something she would say 'well yes, but what about this?' and she made us think a little bit broader than what we were as a team of 5, so I think she was ... I think it was easier with her being there as a facilitator....*
>
> *(Female newly qualified Physio PQ105)*

In addition, the students felt confident to implement different ways of working without fear of reprisal or ridicule.

> *I mean the (real) MDT was good ... and from that we based our (student) MDT at the end of the week on how could we make it better ...*
>
> *(Female Student Physio 07)*

And I think the way we did it...Obviously there were some technical hitches, but I think it did work quite well. Which was pleasing cos we had tried to break everything down and change it from the one we saw on the Monday, to try and improve it. I think some of that came through.

(Female Student Medic E07)

Conclusion

This chapter has covered a practice model of IPE in great detail, providing templates and guidance. There are obviously many other models and we have provided a list of several we are aware of (see also Chapters 3, 5 and 10). Practice based models are different in many ways to online models (Chapter 6), although both approaches offer the same challenges. The interprofessional learning in practice has the advantage of being realistic, applied, in the workplace and owned by frontline practitioners. The logistics and workload required to develop and implement such models should not be underestimated and we recommend that if you are considering going down this road that you read chapter 10 on the collaborative model which we believe provides key elements necessary to develop sustainable IPE, which promotes and encourages students and practitioners at the very least to work cooperatively, but is very likely to promote collaborative working which we believe will result in improved patient care.

Other UK models of interprofessional activities

Anderson, E., N. Manek and A. Davidson. (2006). Evaluation of a model for maximizing interprofessional education in an acute hospital. *Journal of Interprofessional Care* 20: 2, 182–194.

Lindqvist, S., A. Duncan, L. Shepstone, F. Watts and S. Pearce. (2005). Case based learning in cross-professional groups – the development of a pre-registration interprofessional learning programme. *Journal of Interprofessional Care* 19 (5): 509–520.

Parsell, G., R. Spalding and J. Bligh. (1998). Shared goals, shared learning: Evaluation of a multiprofessional course for undergraduate students. *Medical Education* 32: 304–311.

O'Halloran, C., S. Hean, D. Humphris and J. Macleod-Clark. (2006). Developing common learning: The new generation project undergraduate curriculum model. *Journal of Interprofessional Care* 20 (1): 12–28.

Reeves, S. and D. Freeth. (2002). The London training ward: An innovative interprofessional learning initiative. *Journal of Interprofessional Care* 16(1): 41–52.

International models of interprofessional activities

Cook, D.A. (2005). Models of inter professional learning in Canada. *Journal of Interprofessional Care* 19(S1) May: 107–115.
Flemming, J., Anna Marie Fink, Vibeke Marcussen, Kristian Larse, and Torben BæK Hansen. (2009). Interprofessional undergraduate clinical learning: Results from a three year project in a Danish Interprofessional Training Unit. *Journal of Interprofessional Care* 23(1) January: 30–40.
Thistlethwaite, J. and G. Nisbet. (2007). Interprofessional education: What's the point and where we're at... *The Clinical Teacher* 4(2): 67–72.

References

Anderson, E., N. Manek and A. Davidson. (2006). Evaluation of a model for maximizing interprofessional education in an acute hospital. *Journal of Interprofessional Care* 20 (2): 182–194.
Barker, K.K., K. Bosco and I.F. Oandasan. (2005). Factors in implementing interprofessional education and collaborative practice initiatives: Findings from key informant interviews. *Journal of Interprofessional Care* May 19 (Suppl. 1): 166–176.
Bluteau, P.A.S. and J.A. Jackson. (2005). Recycling established patterns of working: A method for implementing inter professional learning. *CAIPE Bulletin* Spring.
D'Eon, M. (2005). A blue print for interprofessional learning. *Journal of Interprofessional Care* 19 May(Suppl. 1): 49–59.
Freeth, D., S. Reeves, C. Goreham, P. Parker, S. Haynes and S. Pearson. (2001). 'Real life' clinical learning on an interprofessional training ward. *Nurse Education Today* 21(5): 366–372.
Gilbert, J.H.V. (2005). Interprofessional learning and higher education structural barriers. *Journal of Interprofessional Care* 19 (Suppl. 1): 87–106.
Jackson, J.A. and P.A.S. Bluteau. (2007). At first it's like shifting sands: Setting up interprofessional learning within a secondary care setting. *Journal of Interprofessional Care* 21(3) June: 351–353.
Lennox, A. and E.S. Anderson. (2007). *The Leicester Model of Interprofessional Education: A Practical Guide to Implementation in Health and Social Care Education.* Special Report 9, The Higher Education Academy Subject Centre for Medicine, Dentistry and Veterinary Medicine.
Lindqvist, S., A. Duncan, L. Shepstone, F. Watts and S. Pearce. (2005). Case based learning in cross-professional groups – the development of a pre-registration interprofessional learning programme. *Journal of Interprofessional Care* 19 (5): 509–520.

O'Halloran, C., S. Hean, D. Humphris and J. Macleod-Clark. (2006). Developing common learning: The new generation project undergraduate curriculum model. *Journal of Interprofessional Care* 20 (1): 12–28.

Reeves, S. and D. Freeth. (2002). The London training ward: An innovative interprofessional learning initiative. *Journal of Interprofessional Care* 16(1): 41–52.

Roschelle, J. and S. Teasley. (1995). The construction of shared knowledge in collaborative problem solving, in O'Malley, C.E. (ed.) *Computer Supported Collaborative Learning*. Heidelberg: Springer-Verlag, pp. 69–97.

6
An e Learning Model of Interprofessional Education

Patricia Bluteau and Ann Jackson

Introduction

This chapter aims to describe one e learning model of interprofessional education (IPE) which occurs virtually across four university sites, innumerable practice placements and on the plethora of computers across the homes of participating students and facilitators. It aims to enable the reader to have an insight into the development, implementation and evaluation of this model. The ideal IPE model, whilst meeting the aims of IPE set out by CAIPE, would also be cost and time efficient. More importantly perhaps, is the need to offer IPE activities which engage all participating students, so that they appreciate the benefits of collaboration and teamworking not only for patients/service users/clients/carers, but also for themselves. These activities need to be sustainable over time. This chapter will look at one model of IPE – an online model interwoven through a three year curriculum, which allows IPE activities to be undertaken asynchronously by large numbers of students (1000+) simultaneously. The advantage of this model is the method of delivery which allows students in any location and on any shift pattern and length to participate in IPE activities – the challenges, however, are IT access with the necessary prerequisites to access and run the software, the lack of face-to-face contact, and the fact that students can work cooperatively as opposed to collaboratively (see Chapter 10).

It is important to mention that online IPE is gathering pace across the UK and further a field with a growing body of evidence helping to create and develop new ways of working in an interprofessional 'virtual' world (Connor, 2003; Hughes *et al.*, 2004; Juntunen and Heikkinen, 2004; Moule, 2006; Miers *et al.*, 2007).

Interprofessional e Learning Pathway (IPeLP)

It is unlikely that any one method of IPE will be perfect – there are those (both student and teacher alike) who are emphatic that IPE has to occur within practice for it to have any learning value; there are others who believe that IPE must also have a base in academic learning if it is to be seen of educational value; and there are those who do not see the need for IPE at all. Blended learning may be the way to satisfy both camps, although IPE in practice is more likely to win over the sceptics.

The IPeLP provides IPE via an online medium, allowing students to explore and discuss topics relevant to their IPE objectives at a very early stage in their training (first term/semester), as well as providing the opportunity to build on learning and understanding, allowing the delivery of increasingly more complex topics/issues at varying points through professional training.

Here we will describe the actual requirements of the pathway as well as the changes over time.

Overall aim of the IPeLP

- To provide students with an understanding of the importance and relevance of the roles and responsibilities of different professional groups involved in delivering patient/client/service user care.
- To embed within the undergraduate curriculum of 13 health and social care professional groups in two higher education institutions.
- To weave IPE throughout each professional curriculum building on and reinforcing learning.

The IPeLP has 3 levels (Table 6.1). Each level lasts 4 weeks. Level 1 begins very early in the participating professionals' entire curriculum (i.e. 2 months following start of their training). Level 2 occurs in year 2 and Level 3 in year 3 of student training. For those professions undertaking a four year course, Level 3 is placed in year 4 of their training.

Table 6.1 Timings of IPeLP

IPeLP levels	Length of online activity	Time of year	Year of training
Level 1	4 weeks	November/December	Year 1
Level 2	4 weeks	May/June	Year 2
Level 3	4 weeks	March/April	Year 3 (4)

Learning outcomes and delivery format

The IPeLP draws on the Interprofessional Capability Framework (CUILU, 2004) for it's learning outcomes at Levels 1, 2 and 3. Each level is supported by a student guide (Appendix 1). Students are expected to complete summative reflective pieces of work which are supported with evidence of their own and their colleagues' contributions to the virtual discussion board. Currently, the IPeLP uses a series of case journeys as a focus for group discussion. Attached to each journey are a series of weekly e-activities which students are expected to complete.

Online IPE provides an environment, where large numbers of students can participate irrespective of placement, institution or type of course (e.g. part time/full time). At each level the IPeLP can cater for over 1000 students participating simultaneously online (Table 6.2).

Students work in virtual learning sets (VLS), of 15, supported by one e-facilitator to two groups. There is usually a student mix of 4–6 professional groups per VLS. Each VLS has their own case journey and their own web-based discussion forum, which is only accessible by members of the group and their facilitator. The facilitator plays an important role in the group discussions by encouraging the students to participate, to diffuse any difficult or stereotypical comments and to answer any questions. All facilitators are trained in interprofessional e-facilitation

Table 6.2 Range of Professional Groups Participating in IPeLP

Professional groups

Occupational therapists	Operating department practitioners	Learning disability nurses
Physiotherapists	Adult nurses	Medics
Social workers	Children nurses	Midwives
Mental health nurses	Dieticians	Paramedics
Clinical psychologists	Youth workers	

skills prior to facilitating, in a five-week course which is based upon the Gilly Salmon (2000) e-facilitation model.

The case journeys are authentic, based on real life experiences, and students are matched to the journey according to its relevance to their discipline. This ensures that all students, within the group, have a role to play in the delivery of care within the journey.

Students are brought together for one face-to-face session prior to completing the 4-week case journey online. This face-to-face session provides students and the facilitator with an opportunity to meet each other and to learn about the course design and learning outcomes of the online patient journey. Organising the face-to-face sessions is a logistical challenge, finding rooms and time when all students are free is difficult; our experience, however, shows that the majority of students prefer to meet prior to the online activity at Level 1; thereafter in Levels 2 and 3, meeting or not meeting prior to the start of the online pathway does not seem to be important or affect student participation.

The online environment

Here the need for a learning technologist is a must. The opening page needs to be engaging and welcoming to both students and facilitators alike (Figure 6.1). It has to provide all the information necessary to

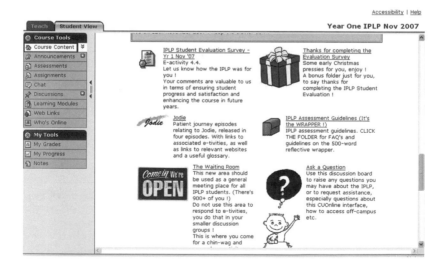

Figure 6.1 Making the online environment interesting and welcoming

complete the pathway (assessment information, student guide, access to individual discussion group and a forum where they can ask any questions), prior to the release of the first episode and following the face-to-face session. It is useful and important that all students access the online forum prior to the start of the online activities. Not only does this identify and provide time to resolve access and log in problems with any students but also allows time for ironing out any navigation difficulties a student may have. This is especially important when the level of computer literacy and ability of each student is unknown.

All students are encouraged to explore the front page of the site and to post a message in the 'Arrivals Lounge'. Students are also able to enter their group discussion forum which has a brief overview of the case journey they will be studying.

In our experiences students particularly value the 'Arrivals Lounge' which they are able to use as a chat line to over 1000 colleagues. Initially, we found it necessary to close the lounge once the first episode was released as it proved to be confusing for some students who tried to complete their small group activities in this larger forum. Prior to the launch of the journey the learning technologist and IPeLP year leads monitor student online activity and answer any difficulties via the 'Ask a Question' thread. This means that most access and navigation difficulties are rectified prior to starting the journey.

Facilitators web space

The creation of a facilitator web space which is 'safe' from students is useful, some would say essential (Figure 6.2). Within this space there are student group lists (with e-mail addresses), essential when trying to make contact with non-participating students.

A virtual café provides refreshments and a chance to share issues with colleagues. A 'Help needed' section provides the opportunity to identify and resolve difficulties. A 'Good tips' provides sharing of best practice between facilitators, especially useful when the course is running. Sharing information in this way shares the workload by providing such things as 'welcome messages', techniques for managing the discussion space and so on.

Case journeys

For Levels 1 and 2, 12 e learning case journeys are available for use. Each year they are reviewed to ensure that they are still accurate. Most of these

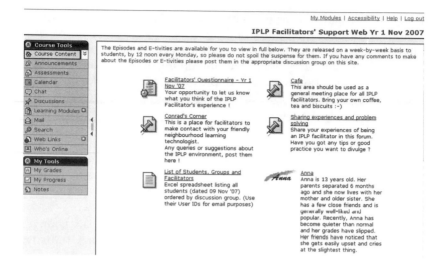

Figure 6.2 Facilitator forum web space on the IPeLP

journeys are authentic and follow a person's journey along a care path-way. These journeys involve a medical condition such as cancer, mental health or in others pregnancy or drug abuse. The journeys are divided into four episodes, each week an 'episode' of the journey is released (Figure 6.3).

Use of video, audio or written text can be used to deliver each weekly episode; currently, we deliver most episodes by written text, as this requires the least sophisticated software and advanced computer for access. We have experienced minimal problems with students access-ing video transcripts (where we have used them) and student feedback has shown that they are welcome additions to each episode providing a 'face' to the journey. The art of each video, however, is to ensure that they are short and specific. Where we have used audio to supplement the journey (these tend to be tapes capturing experienced health and social care professionals' views on their role in the specific case journey), we did experience some problems with this format as many computers out on placement do not have, or have disabled, the audio outlet and where the audio does work students need to have earphones. As we have no way of controlling for this we always provide a transcription of the interview.

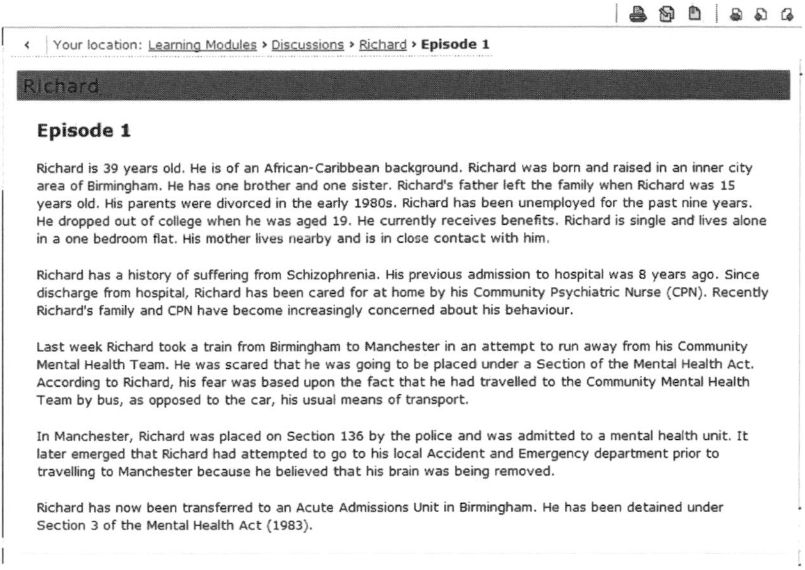

Your location: Learning Modules › Discussions › Richard › **Episode 1**

Richard

Episode 1

Richard is 39 years old. He is of an African-Caribbean background. Richard was born and raised in an inner city area of Birmingham. He has one brother and one sister. Richard's father left the family when Richard was 15 years old. His parents were divorced in the early 1980s. Richard has been unemployed for the past nine years. He dropped out of college when he was aged 19. He currently receives benefits. Richard is single and lives alone in a one bedroom flat. His mother lives nearby and is in close contact with him.

Richard has a history of suffering from Schizophrenia. His previous admission to hospital was 8 years ago. Since discharge from hospital, Richard has been cared for at home by his Community Psychiatric Nurse (CPN). Recently Richard's family and CPN have become increasingly concerned about his behaviour.

Last week Richard took a train from Birmingham to Manchester in an attempt to run away from his Community Mental Health Team. He was scared that he was going to be placed under a Section of the Mental Health Act. According to Richard, his fear was based upon the fact that he had travelled to the Community Mental Health Team by bus, as opposed to the car, his usual means of transport.

In Manchester, Richard was placed on Section 136 by the police and was admitted to a mental health unit. It later emerged that Richard had attempted to go to his local Accident and Emergency department prior to travelling to Manchester because he believed that his brain was being removed.

Richard has now been transferred to an Acute Admissions Unit in Birmingham. He has been detained under Section 3 of the Mental Health Act (1983).

Figure 6.3 Example of year 1 case scenario

Each episode is supported by a series of activities which the students must complete. Usually there are about 3–4 activities although the number is dependent on the content of each activity (Box 6.1).

Box 6.1 e-Activity 1.1: Week 1: IPeLP: Level 1

e-Activity 1.1

Hello and welcome

It's time to meet each other online. The main area for discussion, debate and learning will be in the discussion area which in effect is an online conferencing facility. Whenever you see an e-activity described, you should be able to click on the related discussion area, displayed under 'Discussions', so that you can start contributing straight away.

Aim

To let us know that you have arrived safely post a message into your discussion group.

Box 6.1 (Continued)

Objective

Post a message and tell us who are you, what course you are studying on and what your expectations are of the pathway?

You may like to attach a photograph of yourself to your posting, to allow your group members to put a face to a name! (When creating your message click on 'Enable HTML Creator' to access the HTML Editor which allows you to do great things like adding a picture and using the spell-checker).

Note: If you do manage to attach a photograph to your posting, please assist your colleagues who may not be so technically minded.

If you succeeded in posting a message last week, please expand on your initial thoughts and impressions of the IPeLP.

By episode 3 there may only be 2–3 activities but each activity may have two parts – for example, each student may be asked to describe their own professional role in the case scenario at this point, and to ask a question of one or two other professions in their discussion group. This means that they provide a description of their own role; they ask two questions of the others and have to respond to any questions asked of them (Box 6.2). This sort of activity aims to encourage student exploration of each other and to encourage 'conversation' type postings – if this works (it is highly dependent on the students' motivation to participate and log in frequently), then the students begin to relate to one another and real student interaction can be observed.

Box 6.2 e-Activity 2.2: Week 2: IPeLP: Level 1

e-Activity 2.2

Aim

To explore the role of different professional groups in supporting the family of the patient.

Objective

1. First, read the latest episode and consider the role that your profession would play in both supporting and giving information to the family. If your profession is not involved at this stage, how would you expect other professions to be communicating with you and considering your possible future involvement?

2. Post a considered response to at least two other postings from your colleagues. Once you have completed this task continue with e-activity 2.3.

One of the problems with online groups relates to the asynchronous nature of the medium – that is, some students will complete the activities by Monday (the day they are released) and will be awaiting a response from fellow students, whilst others may not even log in until Thursday/Friday. This delay can be very de-motivating for students and so it is an important aspect to highlight and encourage students to engage at the very beginning of the journey – we have recently introduced a student agreement form which all students sign to agree to log in online at least 3 times per week – it is possible that we will also make this an assessed aspect of the 4 weeks, although it is likely that enforcing this will increase the facilitators' workload. Another difficulty is ensuring (a) that students do complete the second part of the activity and (b) that they respond to any questions posed by their colleagues. It seems that students can quite easily complete the activities yet not be truly interacting – a token exercise. Whilst facilitation can, to some degree, prompt and remind students that there are still some incomplete activities, it is the student who has to be self-motivated enough to want to participate – online learning really is a case of the more you put in, the more you get out. Where students possess this motivation, the online discussions and learning with, from and about each other are rich; where students are not motivated, the result is a superficial but passable example of cooperative behaviour. It is likely that students are still learning with, from and about each other, but it is not openly acknowledged. For us, this is the whole crux of IPE: the need for students to be motivated to work interprofessionally, and whilst facilitators can support this, it is for each student to realise that they have a professional responsibility and duty to learn as much as possible about each other, breaking down as many barriers as possible so that in practice they can work collaboratively as a team to deliver best care to their patients/clients/service users.

Throughout the case journey, students are able to share and discuss their roles and responsibilities in relation to the events occurring in each episode. At the end of each level there is a summatively assessed piece of reflective work.

Annually, the case journeys are sent to each professional group for comments; this allows for changes to be made so that the journeys reflect current practice. With the development of specialist posts within and between professions, this can be quite difficult – for example, many case journeys will involve sub-specialties of medicine – for example, GP, Oncologist, Surgeon and so on – so each one should comment on the role of their specialty in each journey. It is also interesting to observe how quickly the journeys date and pathways change, possibly reflecting the current climate in the National Health Service (NHS). With this in mind new learning objects are being continually developed and placed in the Centre for Interprofessional e learning (CIPeL) learning object repository which can be accessed by obtaining a username and password from the CIPeL website www.cipel.ac.uk.

Student anxieties and concerns

The most common anxieties and concerns expressed by students relate to their understanding and navigating the learning environment. Comparison of the different professional groups reveals a wide age range, different educational levels, competing demands on time – with many students having family commitments and little experience of IT.

Level 1 IPeLP is possibly the greatest challenge in terms of IT competency. With the online activity commencing within 6–8 weeks of enrolment on the course, many students are still confused by virtual environment. It is important, therefore, to ensure that IT training day/drop in sessions are available to students, so that they can be guided through the environment and feel confident in finding their discussion space and able to post their comments.

We have found, however, that irrespective of the amount of drop in sessions available there will always be some students who do not fully understand the environment. Sometimes this can be useful as an ice breaker when other students will respond to a cry for help from fellow colleagues. Subsequent IPeLP runs do not seem to have this problem, by virtue of students being further on in their training and being used to the environment.

We have also found that as Level 1 is situated at the beginning of their training many students are not completely sure of their own professional roles or responsibilities. Whilst some students feel able to share this with their colleagues, others tend to feel that they should know this or worse that students from the other professionals will expect them to know. This can result in extreme anxiety to such an extent that students stop participating online. For example, one student contacted his facilitator to raise such an issue. Talking with the student revealed that he was completely fixated on being able to explain the physiology and anatomical structures associated with a medical condition, instead of drawing on his learning to date, which involved communication skills, breaking bad news and health inequalities – all highly relevant to the particular journey.

Links to relevant sites are available for the students, which can help them fill gaps in their knowledge, and if they are on placement they can, and often do, ask more experienced colleagues any questions relating to their roles and responsibilities.

Whilst students out on placement are able to seek advice of colleagues, as well as observe what happens, there are challenges relating to the time IPeLP takes and where this is to be found – is it tied into the practice hours or does it fall within university hours? We have experienced problems with students working a 40-hour week, not being allowed to have time during their shift to go online and so having to find the time either on their days off or late in the evening. As yet, this remains an unresolved issue.

In relation to computer access in practice there were initial concerns (despite checking) that computers within the NHS would not have the necessary software to run the virtual environment. We have only experienced one trust where the computers seemed to be unable to run the software and this was resolved by use of a flying squad (telephone assistance). It is possible, however, that we have not experienced more problems with access in practice because most students are logging on at home or at the university at the end of a shift.

Assessment

Each level of the pathway is assessed – however, at three universities this assessment is summative, at the other formative. Assessment has a tendency to drive students and this is true of the pathway. The structure and content of the pathway as well as the overall aims lends itself to a reflective piece of work. At Level 1 students are expected to complete a 500-word reflective wrapper which explores their own understanding of their professional roles and responsibilities, is supported by a minimum of three of their own postings from the discussion board, as well as an exploration of one other professional group reference with postings supporting their reflections.

For those students who are classed as unsatisfactory and for whom this is a summative piece of work, there is an opportunity to resubmit once they have completed the extraordinary IPeLP run.

Students, for whom this is a formative piece of work, are advised if their piece of work would have been unsatisfactory, but as they are examined on interprofessional roles and responsibilities at the end of semester exams, there is no need for them to resubmit their work.

Equity across all professional groups in terms of assessment, access and workload has proved to be one of the biggest challenges. We have touched on the assessment being summative and formative, but perhaps a more pressing and volatile issue relates to submission deadlines. Recently due to major differences in student activity within the four universities, one professional group were given a different submission date. The students voiced their thoughts on this using the 'Ask a question' forum open to all students. The ensuing debate was mediated by the learning technologist and IPeLP leads and raised some important issues. We now realise that equity across student groups is essential – without it student prejudices and stereotypes between different professions and universities rise to the surface.

Evaluation

As with every module it is important that evaluation data is collected and used to redefine, shape and build on the scenarios and develop the pathway. Obtaining student feedback seems notoriously difficult especially when it is online. Response rates as low as 27% are not uncommon. A tip to obtain high response rates is to make it an e-activity which all students need to complete – this idea from our learning technologist resulted in response rates of over 80%.

Obtaining feedback of facilitators is just as important but it is impossible to make it an activity – so response rates, for us, tend to be low.

Our online evaluation asks students to rate, on a five-point Likert scale, ranging from strongly disagree to strongly agree, a series of statements. Space is also available for free comments.

Evaluation findings from the Level 1 IPeLP showed that the majority of students (≥80%) agreed that interacting online with other students helped them in their studies. Working with students from other professional groups was also highly valued (≥80%). However, getting the number and pace of e-activities is important, as only 60% agreed that the pace was correct. Using the case journey approach seemed relevant to most students, with 80% agreeing that it was relevant to their studies, as well as being interesting.

Forty per cent of students, however, perceived that the IPeLP did not significantly increase their understanding of their own professional roles and responsibilities, presumably many students felt that they did have a good understanding of their own profession even at this early stage in their career. This observation warrants further investigation given that several authors of evaluation tools have suggested that students at this stage in their training are not sure of their own roles and responsibilities. Against this though, over 80% of students felt that participating in the IPeLP had increased their confidence and provided them with a better understanding of the roles of other professional groups.

Facilitator feedback provides some useful information about how the students respond to the e-activities and how they work as a group. It can also provide important information relating to the amount of administration and managing the online groups and the time spent chasing non-participants. The amount of time spent online was surprisingly less than had been anticipated with most facilitators spending 2–4 hours per week, and accessing the site more than 3 times per week.

Student qualitative comments

I have enjoyed being able to gain information and other peoples view of a patient. Understanding of how important the other health team members our and how we all play important parts in the care of a patient. it worked well online as we got to interact with people via an easy source for people to use.

(4) No 482

I don't feel that I have learnt anything new about the professions. I'm not sure what stage the other students are at, but I feel that I have learnt more from qualified practicing HCP's or from later year students who are in clinical practice placements. I feel that proper IPeLP would be better suited to clinical placements where groups could meet in real MDT meetings to discuss a real patient and compare how they would manage the patient with how they have really been managed.

(1) No 690

It has been interesting to see what other students have to say on any particular matter, however I am not convinced that simply posting messages on a particular topic has been any huge benefit in terms of working as a multi disciplinary team. I think this will come from practical experiences in a clinical setting.

(1) No 108

Facilitator qualitative comments

The highlights were when the students were eventually; talking; to each other and my role as facilitator became less important to the group. When they asked each other questions and researched the answers and then shared their findings, it was a delight. They disciplined themselves reminding each other to adhere to the posting rules. Even students who had to be reminded to maintain a tidy site, they were most polite and compliant. Late comers seemed to work hard to catch up and become involved. No real difficulties managing the groups ... Without a doubt the success depended on the level of student participation. It seems to have worked!

Respondent 1 (07)

I encountered very little difficulty this time except confirming the where-abouts of non-attendees (which got sorted eventually). The highlights were watching the group gel well and take off the discussion themselves with cohesion and respect.

Respondent 16 (07)

Actually far more effective for students than I had anticipated. It was a pleasant surprise to see perceptions and assumptions being chal-lenged/changing in many cases. Students were also obviously surprised about this and often about their ability to access the system. Very hard with students who don't engage or answer your e-mails ... horse to water etc. Also hard on other students who want to interact.

Respondent 12 (07)

I was not looking forward to this when I had finished the e-spire course as I knew that it would add to my already stiff workload. However, I enjoyed it, looked forward to reading the posts and am actually looking forward to the next run.

Respondent 4 (07)

Conclusion

The initial setting up and development of the IPeLP was a significant amount of hard work. Too few people drawn in to develop the envi-ronment at grass roots put huge pressure on those of us who were left to cope, but although concerns were raised in the initial runs regarding the integration of virtual interprofessional learning into uniprofessional curricula it is now embedding and more individuals are keen to claim some allegiance to it. The IPeLP has the advantage that it can be used with a wide range of professional groups, with large numbers of students, irrespective of practice or theoretical placement whilst still being relevant to each student's professional development.

References

Connor, C. (2003) Virtual learning and inter-professional education: Developing computer mediated communication for learning about collaboration. *Innovations in Education and Teaching International.* 40, 341–347.

CUILU (2004) *Interprofessional Capability Framework.* Sheffield: Combined Universities Interprofessional Leaning Unit.

Hughes, M., S. Ventura and M. Dando. (2004) Online interprofessional learning: Introducing contructivism through enquiry based learning and peer review. *Journal of Interprofessional Care.* 18, 263–268.

Juntunen, A. and E. Heikkinen. (2004) Lessons from interprofessional e-learning: Piloting a care of the elderly module. *Journal of Interprofessional Care.* 18, 269–278.

Miers, M.E., B.A. Clarke, K.C. Pollard, C.E. Rickaby, J. Thomas and A. Turtle. (2007) Online interprofessional learning: The student experience. *Journal of Interprofessional Care.* 21(5), 529–542.

Moule, P. (2006) E-learning for healthcare students: Developing the communities of practice framework. *Journal of Advanced Nursing.* 54, 370–380.

Salmon, G. (2000) *E-Moderating: The Key to Teaching and Learning Online.* London: Kogan Page.

Part III

Evaluation Tools

In Part III of the book, three chapters outline validated and tested interprofessional education (IPE) evaluation tools. In Chapter 7, Karen Mattick and John Bligh focus on the Readiness for Interprofessional Learning Scale (RIPLS) which aims to investigate student attitudes towards IPE. It was designed originally for use with undergraduate students and has been used widely (internationally and within UK) and more recently in postgraduate settings as well. RIPLS is appropriate for examining attitudes across groups or across time but was not designed for evaluation of short interprofessional learning (IPL) intervention. Work continues to develop this tool.

In Chapter 8 Sarah Hean builds on John Carpenter's earlier work to focus on the measurement of stereotypes in evaluating IPL and explores why stereotypes warrant exploration and evaluation. The chapter gives advice on when it is appropriate to use and how to use and access the scales. It draws on examples where the scale has been used and touches on the findings. It concludes with an overview of its limitations and gaps in knowledge in relation to stereotypes.

In Chapter 9 Suzanne Lindqvist has completed this part of the book by looking at the questionnaire she has developed; the attitudes to health professionals questionnaire (AHPQ). It provides the reader with a background to the development of the tool, how it relates to IPL and its importance in evaluating IPE. The chapter also outlines how this tool has been used and findings from its use are shared with the reader. These three chapters encourage the reader to explore some of the key evaluation tools available for use in the evaluation of IPE. By bringing these three tools together the reader is able to compare their usage when considering evaluation of IPE in their own settings.

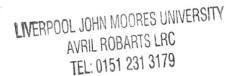

7

Readiness for Interprofessional Learning Scale

Karen Mattick and John Bligh

Introduction

The Readiness for Interprofessional Learning Scale (RIPLS; Parsell and Bligh 1999) is a 19-item self-report inventory, scored using a 5-point Likert scale, which aims to investigate attitudes towards interprofessional learning (IPL). It was designed originally for use with undergraduate healthcare students, but a recent publication (Reid *et al.* 2006) documents its use in a postgraduate population. It is appropriate for comparing attitudes across groups or across times but was not designed for evaluating a short IPL intervention. Since the number of requests to use the scale is increasing exponentially work is ongoing to strengthen the tool. Findings from its use show interesting differences between the attitudes of groups of healthcare professionals. The scale is available from the authors, via the e-resource set up for researchers, using RIPLS, or in the original publication (Parsell and Bligh 1999). This chapter provides a background to the development of RIPLS and its subsequent modification; we will also discuss how RIPLS has been used throughout the world and summarise the key findings of these studies.

Background to Developing the Scale: Why the RIPLS Was Needed

Patient care is nearly always team-based at the point of delivery. This means that, as well as their discipline-specific knowledge and skills, healthcare professionals must be able to work well in a multidisciplinary team. Multidisciplinary teamwork requires an understanding and respect for the work of other healthcare professionals, in addition to good interpersonal and communication skills.

There is a widespread belief that development of the skills and attitudes, necessary to work effectively within a multidisciplinary team, should begin prior to qualification, during the years of undergraduate study. This belief has led to the introduction of a large number of IPL initiatives in undergraduate healthcare programmes over the past two decades.

When one stops to consider the roots of such a belief, there emerges some theoretical basis to support what many feel intuitively is good practice. For example, complex systems theory suggests that in a complex system the sum of the parts (i.e. the individuals within a team) may not be a good approximation of the emergent capability of the whole system (i.e. the team functioning). Similarly, activity theory highlights the social and collaborative aspects of human activity, which can make the difference between a highly functioning team and a less good one.

The empirical evidence in support of IPL, however, has been, and still is, relatively unconvincing (Zwarenstein *et al.* 1999; Mattick and Bligh 2003). Unfortunately, much of the work has been performed at a relatively low level in Kirkpatrick's hierarchy (1994), with evaluations of IPL initiatives tending to focus on participant's satisfaction, rather than targeting difficult to measure but important aspects like attitudinal and behaviour change. But even the well-designed and executed studies have largely failed to demonstrate marked benefits resulting from IPL initiatives.

In this context, it was recognised that a tool to measure temporal changes in attitudes towards IPL could move the debate forward and characterise those aspects of interventions and curricula associated with positive trends. This has the potential to improve patient care, through the provision of undergraduate programmes that promote interdisciplinary teamworking. Thus, in 1998, the scene was set for the development of the RIPLS.

How the RIPLS was developed and evaluated originally

Practitioners that developed and evaluated IPL courses, prior to 1999, reported various characteristics and conditions that were associated with success. Parsell and Bligh (1999) observed that these grouped into four key dimensions (Box 7.1).

Box 7.1 Four Key Dimensions

1. Relationships between different professional groups (values and beliefs people hold);
2. Collaboration and teamwork (knowledge and skills needed);
3. Roles and responsibilities (what people actually do);
4. Benefits to patients, professional practice and personal growth (what actually happens).

Parsell and Bligh (1999) generated a large pool of items reflecting these four dimensions, using literature, expert opinion and personal experience. The items were assessed by 13 experts and rated individually for their relevance to multiprofessional shared learning. The experts also gave feedback about the clarity and format of the items. The resulting scale was completed by a sample of second year degree students across 8 professions ($n = 120$), using a 5-point Likert scale (strongly agree to strongly disagree) to score the items. Principal components analysis was performed with varimax rotation[1] in order to identify items that might be representing a single underlying construct.

Methods for investigating the reliability and validity for questionnaire items were then applied to achieve a staged removal of the less useful items until a 19-item scale (the RIPLS) remained (Table 7.1). The 19-item RIPLS took approximately 8 minutes to complete and had an overall internal consistency (IC, alpha coefficient) of 0.90. It comprised three sub-scales (Table 7.1):

1) 'teamwork and collaboration' (9 items, alpha 0.88) – signifying a belief in the benefits of shared learning, including effective teamworking and relationships with other professionals;
2) 'professional identity' (7 items, alpha 0.63) – relating to both positive and negative aspects of professional identity;
3) 'roles and responsibilities' (3 items, alpha 0.32).

Five items loaded negatively onto the 'teamwork and collaboration' sub-scale, four within the 'professional identity' sub-scale and one within the 'roles and responsibilities' sub-scale.

Table 7.1 Demonstrating the Sub-Scale Structure Reported in Two Publications Subsequent to Parsell and Bligh (1999)

	Parsell and Bligh (1999)	Parsell et al. (1998)	McFadyen et al. (2005)	Bligh and Mattick (unpublished)*	Reid et al. (2006)	El-Zubier et al. (2006)
1 Learning with other students will help me become a more effective member of a healthcare team	Teamwork and collaboration	Teamwork and collaboration	Teamwork and collaboration	Teamwork	Teamwork and collaboration	Teamwork and collaboration
2 Patients would ultimately benefit if healthcare students worked together to solve patient problems	Teamwork and collaboration	Teamwork and collaboration	Teamwork and collaboration	Collaboration	Teamwork and collaboration	–
3 Shared learning with other healthcare students will increase my ability to understand clinical problems	Teamwork and collaboration	Teamwork and collaboration	Teamwork and collaboration	Collaboration	Teamwork and collaboration	Teamwork and collaboration
4 Learning with healthcare students before qualification would improve relationships after qualification	Teamwork and collaboration	Teamwork and collaboration	Teamwork and collaboration	Collaboration	Teamwork and collaboration	Teamwork and collaboration
5 Communication skills should be learned with other healthcare students	Teamwork and collaboration	Teamwork and collaboration	Teamwork and collaboration	Collaboration	Teamwork and collaboration	Teamwork and collaboration

Table 7.1 Continued

6	Shared learning will help me to think positively about other professionals	Teamwork and collaboration	Teamwork and collaboration	Teamwork and collaboration	Collaboration	Teamwork and collaboration	Teamwork and collaboration
7	For small group learning to work, students need to trust and respect each other	Teamwork and collaboration	Teamwork and collaboration	Teamwork and collaboration	Teamwork	Teamwork and collaboration	–
8	Teamworking skills are essential for all healthcare students to learn	Teamwork and collaboration	Teamwork and collaboration	Teamwork and collaboration	Teamwork	Teamwork and collaboration	–
9	Shared learning will help me to understand my own limitations	Teamwork and collaboration	Teamwork and collaboration	Teamwork and collaboration	Teamwork	Teamwork and collaboration	Teamwork and collaboration
10	I don't want to waste my time learning with other healthcare students	Professional identity	–	Positive professional identity	Uniqueness of discipline	–	Professional identity
11	It is not necessary for undergraduate healthcare students to learn together	Professional identity	Teamwork and collaboration	Positive professional identity	Uniqueness of discipline	–	Professional identity
12	Clinical problem-solving skills should only be learned with students from my own department	Professional identity	Negative professional identity	Positive professional identity	Uniqueness of discipline	Sense of professional identity	Professional identity

Table 7.1 Continued

	Parsell and Bligh (1999)	Parsell et al. (1998)	McFadyen et al. (2005)	Bligh and Mattick (unpublished)*	Reid et al. (2006)	El-Zubier et al. (2006)
13 Shared learning with other healthcare students will help me to communicate better with patients and other professionals	Professional identity	Teamwork and collaboration	Negative professional identity	Collaboration	Teamwork and collaboration	Teamwork and collaboration
14 I would welcome the opportunity to work on small-group projects with other healthcare students	Professional identity	Teamwork and collaboration	Negative professional identity	Collaboration	Teamwork and collaboration	Teamwork and collaboration
15 Shared learning will help to clarify the nature of patient problems	Professional identity	Teamwork and collaboration	Negative professional identity	Collaboration	Teamwork and collaboration	Teamwork and collaboration
16 Shared learning before qualification will help me become a better teamworker	Professional identity	Teamwork and collaboration	Positive professional identity	Collaboration	Teamwork and collaboration	Teamwork and collaboration
17 The function of nurses and therapists is mainly to provide support for doctors	Roles and responsibilities	Negative professional identity	Roles and responsibilities	Uniqueness of discipline	Sense of professional identity	Professional identity
18 I'm not sure what my professional role will be	Roles and responsibilities	Roles	Roles and responsibilities	Professional role	–	–

Table 7.1 Continued

		Roles and responsibilities	Negative professional identity	Roles and responsibilities	Uniqueness of discipline	Sense of professional identity	
19	I have to acquire much more knowledge and skills than other healthcare students	Roles and responsibilities			Uniqueness of discipline	Sense of professional identity	–
20	There is little overlap between my future role and that of other healthcare professionals				Uniqueness of discipline	Sense of professional identity	Professional identity
21	I would feel uncomfortable if another healthcare student knew more about a topic than I did				Uniqueness of discipline	Sense of professional identity	–
22	I will be able to use my own judgement a lot in my professional role (professional freedom)				Professional role	–	–
23	Reaching a diagnosis will be the main function of my role (clinical object)				Patient-centredness	–	–
24	My main responsibility as a professional will be to treat my patient (clinical object)				Patient-centredness	–	–
25	I like to understand the patient's side of the problem (patient situation)				Patient-centredness	Patient-centredness	Patient-centredness

Table 7.1 Continued

	Parsell and Bligh (1999)	Parsell et al. (1998)	McFadyen et al. (2005)	Bligh and Mattick (unpublished)*	Reid et al. (2006)	El-Zubier et al. (2006)
26 Establishing trust with my patients is important to me (patient situation)				Patient-centredness	Patient-centredness	Patient-centredness
27 I try to communicate compassion to my patients (patient situation)				Patient-centredness	Patient-centredness	Patient-centredness
28 Thinking about the patient as a person is important in getting treatment right (patient situation)				Patient-centredness	Patient-centredness	Patient-centredness
29 In my profession you need skills in interacting and cooperating with patients (patient situation)				Patient-centredness	Patient-centredness	Patient-centredness

*Additional items proposed to strengthen the original sub-scales called professional identity and roles and responsibilities.

Subsequent to this 'pilot study', a further study of 914 undergraduate students across the years of study, 5 professions and 3 institutions was performed (Parsell *et al.* 1998). One of the 19 items (*'I don't want to waste my time learning with other health care students'*) loaded significantly onto two sub-scales and was removed for the purposes of analysing this second data set (Table 7.1). The resulting 18-item scale had an overall IC of 0.74. There were three sub-scales but these were slightly different from the first study (Parsell and Bligh 1999):

1) 'teamwork and collaboration' (14 items [items 1–9, 11, 13–16, Table 7.1], alpha 0.85) – the original 9 items, plus 5 more that originally represented the positive aspects of professional identity;
2) 'negative professional identity' (2 items, alpha 0.85) – with the positive aspects of professional identity now coming into sub-scale 1;
3) 'roles' (1 item).

Although the questionnaire only explains 42% (Parsell and Bligh 1999) and 48% (Parsell *et al.* 1998) of the variance, the RIPLS does seem to be measuring something important. Even at this stage, however, it was clear that the second and third sub-scales were weaker and less well characterised than the first, and further work to characterise and develop the scale was required.

How the RIPLS has been characterised and developed subsequently

The need to refine the RIPLS still further has been outlined previously (Mattick and Bligh 2006). This is not simply to improve the sub-scale structure and reliability of the scale but as our understanding of IPL has moved on significantly since the RIPLS was developed, it is important to ensure that the scale remains current.

Is the scale still as valid today as it was in 1998 when it was first created? It is not unreasonable to suppose that attitudes to IPL are context-specific but there has been considerable interest in using the RIPLS in contexts other than the original sample population. Is the RIPLS valid for use in the new contexts to which it has been applied? This need is pressing when one considers the demand to use the scale. We are aware of 48 researchers across 6 countries who have, or intended to, perform research using the RIPLS in 2005 (Mattick and Bligh 2005). A translation into Swedish has been performed, and we have had enquiries about a Spanish and a Dutch version. This demand highlights the importance of our own work and that of others to strengthen the RIPLS. The most notable contributions to this process are presented chronologically below.

Hind *et al.* 2003

In this study, the 19-item scale was used with first year, UK under-graduate healthcare students from five groups ($n = 933$). The internal consistency was assessed using Cronbach's alpha test, giving a value of 0.80 for the scale overall. The items were summed to provide an overall score for readiness for IPL. No internal consistency values were given for the sub-scales.

McFadyen *et al.* 2005

In this study, data using the 19-item scale were collected from first year, UK healthcare students on starting their undergraduate studies ($n = 308$). Factor analysis applied to these data showed a relatively poor fit with Parsell and Bligh's model (1999):

1) 'teamwork and collaboration' (15 items [items 1–11 and 13–16], alpha 0.80);
2) 'professional identity' (2 items [12 and 17], alpha 0.21);
3) 'roles and responsibilities' (2 items [18 and 19], alpha 0.40).

These observations prompted further exploration and characterisation of the scale (McFadyen *et al.* 2005). Content analysis of the 19 items was performed by seeing if clinical professionals could agree on the group-ings, in which the items could be placed. This led to a solution with four sub-scales which was identical to the model proposed originally (Parsell and Bligh 1999) but with the 'professional identity' sub-scale divided into 'negative professional identity' and 'positive professional identity', rather than having the negative aspects loaded negatively onto a single scale (Table 7.1).

McFadyen used these four sub-scales, as the basis for a model. The fit of the data to all three existing models was assessed (Parsell *et al.* 1998; Parsell and Bligh 1999; McFadyen *et al.* 2005). The fit of the mod-els was similar. For example, the comparative fit index (CFI) was 0.872 for Parsell and Bligh (1999), 0.877 for Parsell *et al.* (1998) and 0.906 for McFadyen's model (2005), where values > 0.90 or preferably > 0.95 indicate an acceptable fit of the data to the model. A second round of data collection followed, from the same students at the end of their first year ($n = 247$). This also showed a very acceptable fit (CFI 0.942 with McFadyen *et al.* 2005 model).

McFadyen *et al.* 2006

So far, the evaluations of the 19-item RIPLS had focused on internal consistency as a measure of its reliability. In this chapter, the test–retest reliability over one week was investigated with a sample of 65 UK health-care students from a single professional group. The test–retest reliability of items, using weighted kappa, was satisfactory for 17 of the items but unsatisfactory for 2 items within sub-scale 2, items 11 and 12 (*'It is not necessary for undergraduate health care students to learn together'* and *'Clinical problem solving skills can only be learned with students form my own department'*, respectively). The intraclass correlations for the sub-scale totals of sub-scales 1 (teamwork and collaboration), 3 (positive professional identity) and 4 (roles and responsibilities) using McFadyen's model (2005) were all greater than 0.6. The intraclass correlation for sub-scale 2 (negative professional identity) was lower at 0.38, containing items 11 and 12 as two of the three items, and deemed unacceptable. Thus sub-scale 2 had a low test–retest reliability in this population of 65 students, although the internal consistency of the sub-scale, as determined previously, was satisfactory (McFadyen *et al.* 2005).

Reid *et al.* 2006

In an effort to strengthen the second and third sub-scales of the original model (professional identity, and roles and responsibilities), Bligh and Mattick, in 2003, proposed ten additional items, derived from the literature and personal experience that they felt might add to the debate and development of the scale (Table 7.1). Since they did not have a multiprofessional sample with which to collect data and evaluate the new items at that time, the new items were made available to other researchers through their e-resource (Mattick and Bligh 2005). The idea was that researchers, who chose to collect data against all the 29 items, could analyse the data with respect to the published 19-item model and the proposed 29-item model.

Reid *et al.*'s study (2006) was the first to publish data associated with the new items. This was also the first study to publish using the RIPLS in a post-qualification population in the UK. A multiprofessional group of qualified healthcare postgraduate tutors considered all the 29 items (the 19 original and 10 new ones) and felt they all had face and content validity. They modified the wording of some items, to reflect the postgraduate context and to include four demographic questions, and delivered the questionnaire, receiving 546 replies. They analysed the data using PCA and varimax rotation, and decided there were 3 sub-scales, using 23 of the items (Table 7.1) and explaining 44.3% of the variance:

1) 'Teamwork and collaboration' (13 items, alpha 0.88);
2) 'Patient-centredness' (5 items, alpha 0.86);
3) 'Sense of professional identity' (5 items, alpha 0.69).

The roles and responsibilities sub-scale did not emerge in this analysis.

El-zubier *et al.* 2006

This study represents the first published use of RIPLS in a non-Western education setting. The 29-item RIPLS was used with senior medical ($n = 90$) and nursing ($n = 88$) students in the United Arab Emirates. The data were analysed using PCA and varimax rotation, with loadings of > 0.4 being considered to make a significant contribution. Items loading onto more than one sub-scale were removed. The overall internal consistency for the scale was 0.61. There were 3 main sub-scales comprising 20 items, together explaining 44% of the variance:

1) 'Teamwork and collaboration' (10 items, alpha 0.86);
2) 'Professional identity' (5 items, alpha 0.80);
3) 'Patient-centredness' (5 items, alpha 0.80).

The teamwork and collaboration and patient-centredness sub-scales were similar to that predicted (Mattick and Bligh 2003) and observed (Reid *et al.* 2006). Whilst both containing 5 items, the professional identify sub-scale of El-zubier *et al.* (2006) and Reid *et al.* (2006) only contained 3 items in common (Table 7.1). Again, the roles and responsibilities sub-scale did not emerge.

What research using the RIPLS has shown

Table 7.2 summarises the key findings of the studies performed to date. In the light of the ongoing evaluation of items and sub-scales, we felt

Table 7.2 Key Findings of Studies Across Professional Groups Using the RIPLS

Authors	Sample population	Tool(s) used	Response rate	Key findings
Horsburgh *et al.* (2001)	First year medicine, nursing and pharmacy students at University of Auckland, New Zealand	19-item RIPLS	180 (90%)	The majority of students reported positive attitudes to shared learning. Nursing and pharmacy students agreed more strongly that learning together would result in more effective teamworking. Medical students were the least sure of their professional role and believed they required more knowledge and skills than nursing or pharmacy students. There were possible gender differences in the responses of students to items
Hind *et al.* (2003)	First year undergraduate healthcare students from five groups (dietetics, nursing, pharmacy, physiotherapy and medicine) in a UK university	19-item RIPLS plus Health Care Stereotypes Scale and Professional Identity Scale	517/933 (55%)	Significant positive correlations between stereotypes, professional identity and readiness for interprofessional learning. Students were positive towards interprofessional learning
Morison *et al.* (2004)	Convenience sample of 20 fourth year medical and 10 third year nursing students in Belfast	19-item RIPLS with additional open questions	n/a	Both groups had strong sense of their professional role. Both perceived IPE as disadvantageous if it impeded their own professional learning

Table 7.2 Continued

Authors	Sample population	Tool(s) used	Response rate	Key findings
Reid et al. (2006)	All GPs, nurses, pharmacists and allied health professionals (AHPs) in Dundee Local Healthcare Co-operation	29-item RIPLS	546/799 (68%)	The mean score on teamwork and collaboration was significantly lower in GPs than in nurses and AHPs. The pharmacists score was significantly lower on patient-centredness than nurses, GPs and AHPs. The GPs score was significantly higher on sense of professional identity than nurses and AHPs
Elzubier et al. (2006)	Senior medical and nursing students at United Arab Emirates University and Institute of Nursing	29-item RIPLS	178/195 (91%)	Both groups were positive about the benefits of undergraduate IPE. 9/10 items in sub-scale 1 were scored significantly higher by nursing students. Three statements in sub-scale 2 were scored significantly lower by nursing students (i.e. they agreed less strongly with items 10, 17, 20 than medical students). Nursing students scored the following statement significantly higher than medical students: 'I try to communicate compassion to my patients.'

it would be inappropriate to present a detailed analysis of the differences between professional groups uncovered through studies using the RIPLS. However, we wish to summarise the main findings to show the potential applications for a robust tool. The initial glimpses are of some interesting differences between the attitudes of groups of healthcare professionals.

Future work required

Summarising the published literature, with respect to the development of the RIPLS and its use with healthcare professionals, has been an interesting exercise on a number of levels. One striking observation is the discrepancy between the number of researchers using, or intending to use, the RIPLS and the number of published papers. It may be that there are a large number of studies in the pipeline, in which case we can expect a bumper crop of publications in the coming year or so. An alternative is that much of the work will never reach the published journals. The latter is a concern we have raised previously (Mattick and Bligh 2003; Mattick and Bligh 2006).

A second observation is the ongoing use of the combination of approaches within exploratory factor analysis termed the 'little jiffy' (Preacher and MacCallum 2003) – namely principal components analysis, retaining components with eigenvalues greater than 1, and using varimax rotation. Using principal components is not compatible with exploring correlations among measured variables (Preacher and MacCallum 2003) – but surely we are interested in correlations between the items in the RIPLS scale. Similarly, varimax is an example of an orthogonal rotation method and as such ensures that the factors do not correlate – but surely we should anticipate some correlation between the sub-scales of the RIPLS and be interested in what this means. And there is little evidence to support (and some to refute) the approach of retaining factors with eigenvalues greater than 1 (Preacher and MacCallum 2003). Therefore, it is important to consider and justify the choices we make within the process of factor analysis and keep up to date with 'best practice' in the methodologies we are using (Mattick and Bligh 2006).

A third observation is that the wording of one of the items has changed slightly in the scale over time from '*It is not necessary for undergraduate health care students to learn together*' (Parsell *et al.* 1998; Parsell and Bligh 1999; Horsburgh *et al.* 2001; McFadyen *et al.* 2005) to

'*It is not beneficial for undergraduate health care students to learn together*' (El-zubier *et al*. 2006, and our latest unpublished work). Whilst on the face of it, this is a minor change, it will be important to monitor the implications of it.

A final, reassuring observation was that a significant number of healthcare professionals have scrutinised the RIPLS items as part of three different studies and consistently conclude there is face and construct validity to them (Parsell and Bligh 1999; McFadyen *et al*. 2005; Reid *et al*. 2006). Therefore, we do believe the RIPLS is tapping something important.

The findings of studies using the 19-item RIPLS reveal a scale with a single strong sub-scale (teamwork and collaboration), and two, or possibly three, much weaker sub-scales. The roles and responsibilities sub-scale had low internal consistency scores in all three studies (Parsell *et al*. 1998; Parsell and Bligh 1999; McFadyen *et al*. 2005) and must be treated with extreme caution, the values for internal consistency being too low to be acceptable for making statements or drawing conclusions.

After the 10 new items were introduced, studies using the 29-item RIPLS have reported three similar sub-scales (Reid *et al*. 2006; El-zubier *et al*. 2006). The internal consistencies of the sub-scales have been encouraging and the items and sub-scales appear to have good face and content validity (Reid *et al*. 2006). These studies also introduced new contexts (postgraduate and non-Western), however, and we have not yet seen published data reporting the same structure in a Western, undergraduate context, in which the RIPLS was originally developed.

In terms of future work needed for the development of the scale, studies with a large population of students across the healthcare discipline in different contexts (but particularly in a Western, undergraduate population) will be important to verify the stability of the three sub-scale structure that has emerged in the latest studies (teamwork and collaboration, professional identity, patient-centredness; Reid *et al*. 2006; El-zubier *et al*. 2006).

If the new three sub-scale structure does prove stable, we will need to consider the implications of having lost the 'roles and responsibilities' aspect of the scale. In one way, this is pleasing since that sub-scale was proving extremely troublesome! If professional perceptions of roles and responsibilities are still deemed an important part of a readiness for IPL, however, then we might need to revisit that aspect of the RIPLS. This might involve generating a large number of items relating to roles and responsibilities, collecting data relating to these items, and seeing if these items load onto the existing sub-scales or form something separate and distinct. As we mentioned earlier, the RIPLS was originally developed in 1998, so it will also be important to ensure that the scale remains current – today's conceptions of IPL are different to those ten years ago. We anticipate that qualitative approaches could have an important role to play in elucidating these two aspects.

The interest in applying RIPLS to contexts, other than those for which it was originally intended, is exciting but these new applications must be properly validated. These include the translations of RIPLS into different languages, its use in other cultures and with qualified healthcare professionals, and for researchers wishing to evaluate a short IPL intervention using a pre- and post-design.

Once the scale is sufficiently robust for use in this way, it will be fascinating to see the differences between professional groups and how readiness for IPL may change over time. But, when using a scale such as the RIPLS, it is important not to get lost in the detail of the methodology but to revisit the bigger questions frequently (Box 7.2).

Box 7.2 Questions Concerning IPL

What is IPL about?

What do learners learn in IPL initiatives?

Is this the same across all learners?

What is the role of attitudes in IPL?

How does the current study contribute to that bigger picture?

It is our belief that engaging with these 'high level' questions will improve the rigour and impact of research using the RIPLS.

We would welcome dialogue about any aspect of this chapter. The scale is available from the authors or in the original publication (Parsell and Bligh 1999).

Note

1. (a combination now largely discredited for this purpose and referred to as the 'little jiffy', Preacher and MacCallum 2003).

References

El-Zubier, M., D.E.E. Rizk and R.K. Al-Khalil. (2006). Are senior UAE medical and nursing students ready for interprofessional learning? Validating the RIPL scale in a Middle Eastern content. *Journal of Interprofessional Care* 20, 619–632.

Hind, M., I. Norman, S. Cooper, E. Gill, R. Hilton, P. Judd and S.C. Jones. (2003). Interprofessional perceptions of health care students. *Journal of Interprofessional Care* 17, 21–34.

Horsburgh, M., R. Lamdin and E. Williamson. (2001). Multiprofessional learning: The attitudes of medical, nursing and pharmacy students to shared learning. *Medical Education* 35, 876–883.

Kirkpatrick, D.L. (1994). *Evaluating Training Programs: The Four Levels.* San Francisco, CA: Berrett-Koehler.

Mattick, K. and J. Bligh. (2003). Interprofessional learning involving medical students or doctors. *Medical Education* 37, 1008–1011.

Mattick, K. and J. Bligh. (2005). An e-resource to coordinate research activity with the Readiness for Interprofessional Learning Scale (RIPLS). *Journal of Interprofessional Care* 19 (6), 604–613.

Mattick, K. and J. Bligh. (2006). Getting the measure of interprofessional learning. Commentary. *Medical Education* 40, 399–400.

McFadyen, A.K., V. Webster, K. Strachan, E. Figgins, H. Brown and J. Mckechnie. (2005). The readiness for interprofessional learning scale: A possible more stable sub-scale model for the original version of RIPLS. *Journal of Interprofessional Care* 19, 595–603.

McFadyen, A.K., V.S. Webste and W.M. Maclaren. (2006). The test-retest reliability of a revised version of the Readiness for Interprofessional Learning Scale (RIPLS). *Journal of Interprofessional Care* 20, 633–639.

Morison, S., M. Boohan, M. Moutray and J. Jenkins. (2004). Developing pre-qualification inter-professional education for nursing and medical students: Sampling student attitudes to guide development. *Nurse Education in Practice* 4, 20–29.

Parsell, G. and J. Bligh. (1999). The development of a questionnaire to assess the readiness of health care students for interprofessional learning (RIPLS). *Medical Education* 33, 95–100.

Parsell, G., A. Stewart and J. Bligh. (1998). Testing the validity of the 'Readiness for Inter-Professional Learning Scale' (RIPLS). Paper presented at the 8th Ottawa International Conference, Philadephia, Pennsylvania.

Preacher, K.J. and R.C. MacCallum. (2003). Repairing Tom Swift's factor analysis machine. *Understanding Statistics* 2, 13–43.

Reid, R., D. Bruce, K. Allstaff and D. McLernon. (2006). Validating the Readiness for Interprofessional Learning Scale (RIPLS) in the postgraduate context: Are health care professionals ready for IPL? *Medical Education* 40, 415–422.

Zwarenstein, M., J. Atkins, H. Barr, M. Hammick, I. Koppel and S. Reeves. (1999). A systematic review of interprofessional education. *Journal of Interprofessional Care* 13, 417–424.

8

The Measurement of Stereotypes in the Evaluation of Interprofessional Education

Sarah Hean

Introduction

This chapter is directed at evaluators using student stereotypes of health and social care (HSC) professionals to understand the processes and outcomes of interprofessional education (IPE) programmes. The chapter focuses on the definition of stereotypes and justifies their inclusion in an evaluation from a theoretical, evaluative and curriculum perspective. This is followed by a summary and discussion of existing means of measurement used in IPE and some practical implications to this endeavour. The chapter concludes with the findings of some existing evaluations.

What are Stereotypes?

Stereotypes are 'social categorical judgment(s)...of people in terms of their group memberships' (Turner, 1999:26). These can be negative judgements leading to prejudiced behaviours towards other social groups (the outgroup). Negative stereotypes may generate false or negative expectations of the outgroup which may become reality through processes of self-fulfilling prophecy (Hilton and von Hippel, 1996). For example, other HSC professionals may stereotype doctors as poor team players. Their interpretation of an individual doctor's actual behaviours may subsequently be coloured by these expectations (Hean *et al.*, 2006a). Negative expectations also have an impact on the target's self-image and output. Negative perceptions in public stereotyping of nursing, for example, may influence the development of poor collective self-esteem, job satisfaction and performance in these professionals (Takase *et al.*, 2002).

Stereotyping, as a natural human process, is not always a negative activity (Haslam *et al.*, 2002). Individuals may use their established stereotypes as a valid mechanism, whereby they make sense of their interactions with other groups with minimum energy expenditure (Haslam *et al.*, 2000; Haslam *et al.*, 2002). In the health arena, specifically, the generalised and often accurate views practitioners hold of a particular patient group may guide them in an appropriate manner when facing an individual from this patient group for the first time (Kirkham *et al.*, 2002; Hean *et al.*, 2006a).

If stereotype use and formation is natural, it is anticipated that HSC students will hold both positive and negative stereotypes of other HSC professional groups. These may be learnt through their own experience of these groups (e.g. as a patient), vicariously (e.g. through the media) (Hallam, 2000; Conroy *et al.*, 2002) or through the socialisation processes, that is professional training (Du Toit, 1995).

Why use stereotypes in IPE evaluation?

If HSC students hold stereotypes of other professional groups, why specifically should these be measured in IPE evaluations and changes monitored over the programme's duration? This question can be answered at a theoretical, evaluative and curricula level.

A theoretical perspective

It has been argued that IPE programmes should be introduced early into students' undergraduate programmes to combat negative stereotypes before these develop or become ingrained (Leaviss, 2000). However, more in-depth theoretical justification is found through consideration of the contact hypothesis and social identity theory.

Contact hypothesis

Stereotype change is a central component of the contact hypothesis. This theory was translated into the IPE arena by Carpenter and colleagues (Hewstone *et al.*, 1994; Carpenter, 1995b, 1995a; Carpenter and Hewstone, 1996; Barnes *et al.*, 2000; Carpenter *et al.*, 2003). It provides practical solutions to overcoming prejudice between different social groups and maintains that positive change in intergroup attitudes will be promoted through encouraging conflicting groups to interact with one another (Allport, 1979). However, interactions must be governed by a set of conditions which include that groups have common goals, are aware of group similarities and differences and that interactions take place within a positive and cooperative atmosphere (Brown *et al.*, 1986; Hewstone and Brown, 1986; Barnes *et al.*, 2000).

IPE provides an opportunity for students of different professional groups to interact under controlled conditions that are conducive to positive changes in their intergroup stereotypes (e.g. Barnes *et al.*, 2000; Carpenter *et al.*, 2003). This may influence the way HSC professionals will interact in the future.

Social identity theory

Group interactions are governed by more than one group simply holding negative/positive stereotypes of another. Intergroup comparisons are also important. Social identity is the identification of self in terms of one's own social group (ingroup) rather than of another group (outgroup) (Turner, 1999). In IPE, the social group in question is the professional group and it is assumed students derive a definition of self from their membership of a particular professional group. When students of different professions interact, they may make comparisons and draw distinctions between the characteristics of their ingroup (autostereotypes) and those of other HSC groups (heterostereotypes) (Tajfel *et al.*, 1971; Carpenter, 1995b, 1995a; Barnes *et al.*, 2006). This comparison is called intergroup differentiation (Tajfel *et al.*, 1971). On the one hand, if students fail to see their group as distinctive, then competitiveness and poor group interrelations result (Branscombe *et al.*, 1999; Zárate and Garza, 2002). On the other hand, some perceived similarities between HSC groups may be desirable as these develop feelings of empathy and a sense of common identification (Stephan and Stephan, 1984; Pettigrew, 1997; Hean *et al.*, 2006b). An appreciation of both similarities and differences between professional groups is recognised as a necessary condition of contact and stereotype change during IPE initiatives (Barnes *et al.*, 2000).

An evaluation perspective

In addition to the theoretical justification for choosing stereotypes in an evaluation, it can also be justified in terms of the evaluation model chosen. Several evaluation models exist but it is largely an adaptation of the Kirkpatrick's evaluation model that has found favour in IPE evaluations (Freeth *et al.*, 2002; Carpenter *et al.*, 2003). This focuses on educational *outcomes* of IPE. At a micro-level, student reactions to IPE and change in their attitudes/knowledge/skills/behaviours are evaluated. At a macro-level, the impact of IPE on the organisation, in terms of improved cross agency communication, working and referral and the benefits accrued to clients are considered (Kirkpatrick, 1967; Allport, 1979; Freeth *et al.*, 2002). Stereotypes and stereotype change are part of the micro-level of analysis and a representation of student attitude/perceptual change.

A curriculum perspective

Evaluators may choose to measure stereotype change because this is an explicit learning outcome of the IPE curriculum. Curricula delivered to undergraduate medical, nursing and social work students (Hewstone *et al.*, 1994; Carpenter, 1995b; Carpenter and Hewstone, 1996) and members of community mental health teams (Barnes *et al.*, 2000; Carpenter *et al.*, 2003) are examples of where the contact hypothesis, and putting in place conditions necessary for stereotype change, are the cornerstone around which IPE curricula have developed. Stereotype change naturally formed part of the evaluation strategies of these programmes.

Stereotype change need not be the key focus of the curriculum for stereotype change still to be relevant. A common learning curriculum (O'Halloran *et al.*, 2006) offered to undergraduate HSC students, for instance, mentions stereotypes only tangentially in the objectives, stating that HSC undergraduate students should develop an 'understanding (of) interprofessional practice...by looking at professional roles and stereotypes and the composition of health and social care teams' (O'Halloran *et al.*, 2006:11). Stereotype measurement still formed part of this programme's evaluation (Hean *et al.*, 2006a; Hean *et al.*, 2006b), the inclusion of this variable being justified along theoretical and evaluation lines.

Ways in which stereotypes can be measured

As the rationale to evaluate student stereotypes may vary, so too may the ways in which stereotypes are measured. For instance, an evaluator may measure students' ratings of:

- overall attitude towards a professional group;
- HSC professional groups on a range of specific characteristics;
- confidence in their ratings of a group on a range of stereotypical characteristics;
- the importance of a range of stereotypical characteristics;
- their propensity to stereotype a group on these characteristics.

The latter three approaches are less well developed, although they represent an attempt to account for the complexity of this domain.

Overall attitude to another professional group

A generic slant to stereotype measurement sees students rating their overall attitude towards another professional group on 7- (Carpenter, 1995b; Carpenter and Hewstone, 1996) or 5-point scales (Tunstall-Pedoe et al., 2003) (Table 8.1).

This is a general affective measure of the student's feelings towards a professional group. Evaluators need to be clear whether they are measuring students' stereotypes of a professional group as a whole (Table 8.1) or if attitudes towards a group of students undergoing particular professional training is the focus. It is conceivable that if it is the former, stereotype change may be harder to achieve than if attitudes to the student group are monitored.

Ratings of specific characteristics

Fishbein and Ajzen (1975) in seminal writing on relationships between attitudes, beliefs and behaviours propose that an individual's overarching attitude to an object is developed from an amalgamation of a series of beliefs they hold of this object. Students' overall attitude towards a professional group will, therefore, be developed through the combination of their beliefs about it. In accordance, a second approach to

Table 8.1 Measurement of Overall Attitude to Professional Group (Carpenter, 1995b; Carpenter and Hewstone, 1996)

My overall attitude to *social workers* is:						
Strongly positive						Strongly negative
1	2	3	4	5	6	7
☐	☐	☐	☐	☐	☐	☐

measuring stereotypes considers these individual beliefs by asking students to rate professional groups on a set of specific characteristics. Likert, semantic differential and visual analogue scales may be used to record these ratings.

Likert scales

Carpenter (1995a) (Box 8.1) generated a list of characteristics perceived by students as typical of nurses and doctors. Final year medical and nursing students rated professional groups on this list using a 7 point Likert scale ranging from very high to very low. This list has subsequently been employed with first year student doctors, pharmacists, dieticians, physiotherapists and nurses (Hind *et al.*, 2003) and with first year student doctors, radiographers, physiotherapists and nurses (Tunstall-Pedoe *et al.*, 2003).

An alternative list of characteristics or part thereof (Boxes 8.2, 8.3 and 8.4) have been employed by other authors (Carpenter and Hewstone, 1996; Barnes *et al.*, 2000; Carpenter *et al.*, 2003). This list is less generic and more specific to the workplace (e.g. autonomy and leadership). Characteristics are presented in a neutral format if compared to the overtly positive/negative adjectives in Box 8.1. For example, students rate communication skills of a professional group (Box 8.3) rather than rating the group as good communicators (Box 8.1). These items have been employed with final year medical and social work students (Box 8.2) as well as qualified members of community mental health teams (psychiatrists, psychologists, nurses, social workers) participating in a career development IPE programme (Boxes 8.3 and 8.4).

Box 8.1 List of Stereotyped Characteristics Used with Undergraduate Students (Carpenter, 1995a)

1. Detached
2. Good communicators
3. Confident
4. Do-gooders
5. Dedicated
6. Arrogant
7. Caring
8. Dithering

Box 8.2 List of Characteristics Used with Final Year
Undergraduate Students (Carpenter and Hewstone, 1996)

1) Breadth of life experience
2) Professional competence
3) Academic quality

Box 8.3 List of Characteristics Used with Qualified HSC
Professionals (Barnes *et al.*, 2000)

1. Academic rigour
2. Breadth of life experience
3. Communication skills
4. Interpersonal skills (e.g. warmth, sympathy, communication)
5. Leadership
6. Practical skills
7. Professional competence

Box 8.4 List of Characteristics Used with Qualified HSC
Professionals (Carpenter *et al.*, 2003)

1. Academic rigour
2. Communication skills
3. Decisiveness
4. Interpersonal skills
5. Leadership
6. Practical skills
7. Professional autonomy
8. Professional competence
9. Team player

Finally, an adaptation of scales described in Boxes 8.2, 8.3 and 8.4 was utilised by Hean *et al.* (2006a) (Box 8.5) to collect baseline data from first year student doctors, midwives, nurses, pharmacists, physiotherapists, occupational therapists, audiologists, social workers and radiographers.

The validity and reliability of these measures, as used originally with qualified professionals was questioned. Students near the end of their training (Carpenter, 1995b, 1995a) or at a postgraduate level (Carpenter *et al.*, 2003) are already familiar with other HSC professionals through placement or work experience. They are likely to have established views on the attributes of other professional groups. This form of measurement may not be appropriate for first year students who do not have the knowledge of the roles, responsibilities or skills of their own, let alone other professionals. Less experienced students' views may therefore be more transient. This may influence the reliability of data they give at the baseline stage of an evaluation (Hean *et al.*, 2003). Hence, items in Box 8.5 were piloted in a panel of academic, HSC practitioners and early undergraduate students of all the participating professions. This validated the format, language and content of the instrument for the lesser educational level and vocabulary of undergraduate students and for the wide number of professional groups involved.

Box 8.5 List of Characteristics with First Year Undergraduate Students (Hean *et al.*, 2006a; Hean *et al.*, 2006b)

1. Academic ability
2. Professional competence
3. Interpersonal skills (e.g. warmth, sympathy, communication)
4. Leadership abilities
5. The ability to work independently
6. Practical skills
7. Confidence
8. The ability to be a team player
9. The ability to make decisions

Piloting showed that students at this level preferred the neutral and work based characteristics (Boxes 8.3 and 8.4) over the value-laden, generic adjectives in Box 8.1. Students displayed resistance to the stereotype questions generally, however, seeing these as an explicit request to stereotype other professional groups. They saw this as contrary to the ethos of IPE (Hean *et al.*, 2003). These reactions may be particular to undergraduate or younger students, more idealistic or less hardened to the 'reality' of poor working relations. Their resistance may be minimised by not using the word *stereotype* explicitly in instructions within a questionnaire and replacing this with the less confrontational *opinion* or *attitude*. Using the more neutral format for questions (see Boxes 8.2, 8.3, 8.4 and 8.5) may also cause less resistance than if the more value-laden adjectives are employed.

Students' reactions to stereotype questions should not be wasted, as facilitators may use these to help students reflect and explore their own and others' preconceptions of other professions and answer questions such as, 'What are the actual characteristics and roles of a profession? Are different values placed on these different characteristics and roles' (Hean *et al.*, 2006a) and, 'How might our attitudes of other HSC professionals influence intergroup working behaviours?'

The stability of responses to items in Box 8.5 was tested over a 2-week period and those that were not reliable over time at a 5% level were removed. Most items were of an acceptable reliability and were transferred directly from the original scale (Barnes *et al.*, 2000). Items, however, where difficulties were observed were adjusted or removed. For example, the characteristic 'breadth of life experience' showed a lack of stability. This may be because students, early in their careers, with limited experience of other professions and professional placement, have not recognised life experience as a relevant attribute or one on which they have any form of established opinion. The most reliable stereotype questions were those items on academic ability. If it is assumed that item stability stands as proxy for a well-formed opinion, it may be hypothesised that consistent views have formed on this academic ability, because students have recently completed a selection procedure to enter the university based almost entirely on their academic performance at A-level. The least reliable items related to the ability of the professional to work independently and professional competence. These professional attributes are further removed from neophyte students' potential field of direct experience and hence produce less reliable responses (Hean *et al.*, 2003).

Semantic differential and visual analogue scales

Other characteristics on which professional groups have been rated in the IPE literature can be viewed in Table 8.2 and Lindqvist *et al.* (2005). Like the characteristics in Table 8.1, these characteristics appear more generic with a lesser professional focus. Mandy *et al.* (2004), for example, measured stereotypes, by asking first year physiotherapy and podiatry students to rate their agreement with a range of opposing adjectives presented in a semantic differentials format (Table 8.2).

A similar approach uses 10 cm visual analogue scale to record ratings (Lindqvist *et al.*, 2005) (see Chapter 9). Undergraduate students rated a range of professionals including social workers, general practitioners and occupational therapists. A more detailed discussion of this measurement tool can be seen in Chapter 9.

Table 8.2 Sample of Bipolar Adjectives Used with Undergraduate Students (Mandy *et al.*, 2004)

Sociable						Exclusive
1	2	3	4	5	6	7
Strong						Weak
1	2	3	4	5	6	7
Interpersonal						Impersonal
1	2	3	4	5	6	7
Attractive						Repulsive
1	2	3	4	5	6	7

Which scale to choose?

No study has explicitly compared and contrasted the benefits of one form of stereotype measurement over another. Until this occurs, the choice of measurement relies on evaluators' own judgement in which a match between a measurement and the particular IPE context is made. Evaluators should consider their own student context and decide whether:

- the instrument has been validated with students of the same educational level (e.g. first year, final year, qualified professionals);
- the instrument has been validated with students of the same professional group;
- the characteristics rated are applicable to their own evaluation. Are perceptions of more generic characteristics such as caring, detached, arrogant (Box 8.1, Table 8.2 and Lindqvist *et al.*, 2005) more likely to be changed by the IPE curriculum or are the more professionally based characteristics (e.g. professional competence, the ability to work independently [Boxes 8.2–8.5 and Table 8.2]) more relevant?
- other studies have used this form of measurement, in order that the findings of their evaluation may be directly compared and contrasted with others in the field.

Importance of each characteristic being measured

IPE studies have concentrated almost entirely on simple ratings of a professional group on a range of specific characteristics. However, stereotypes are not unidimensional constructs. Carpenter *et al.* (2003), for instance, consider a second dimension: the *importance* students place on each characteristic. Stereotypes of characteristics perceived as more important may have a greater effect on intergroup interactions than characteristic assumed to be less so. Carpenter *et al.* (2003) found that students rated interpersonal skills, professional skills and being a team player as most important, and academic rigour and leadership skill as least important.

Propensity to stereotype

Hewstone *et al.* (1994) also recognised the multidimensional dimension of stereotypes. They included in their evaluation, measures of confidence with which stereotypes are held. If more positive stereotypes are reported with greater confidence, this was perceived as a positive outcome of the programme. Subsequently, a further stereotype dimension was identified, the dimension of *perceived variability* (Hewstone and Hamberger, 2000; Hean *et al.*, 2003). This is the degree to which students perceive a professional group to be homogeneous on a particular stereotyped characteristic. For example, students may rate nurses highly on being *caring*. However, if asked to what percentage of nurses this high rating applies, they may believe that whilst the vast majority of nurses are caring (say 75%), there are a significant minority (25%) that are not. The inclusion of this dimension has potential to alleviate students' resistance to stereotype measurement, by enabling them to express the degree they believe a characteristic applies to the group as a whole (Hean *et al.*, 2003). This stereotype dimension still needs to be fully explored in the IPE arena.

Practical challenges in measuring stereotypes

Apart from the choice to be made on which scale or dimension to use, there are also some practical challenges to stereotype measurement. The first relates to the questionnaire format.

Formatting of questions

As the relevance of IPE becomes more recognised in HSC training, a greater diversity of student professional groups become part of these programmes. When only two or three professional groups participate, an evaluation questionnaire in which students rate each of these groups (Carpenter, 1995b) on a range of 8 to 10 characteristics is achievable. This becomes less feasible when 9 or more are part of the evaluation (Hean *et al.*, 2006a, 2006b). If each student is asked to rate each of the nine professional groups, on every characteristic then a long-winded survey, conducive to pattern answering and fatigue, is created.

Some approaches to combating the challenge are to:

- only measure overall attitude to each of the many professional groups involved;
- ask students to rate only a select number of professional groups on the full range of characteristics, selecting those groups about whom the evaluator judges students to have the clearest knowledge (say doctors and nurses), omitting less well-known professionals (say podiatrists and audiologists);
- utilise the format of questionnaire in Table 8.3 (Carpenter *et al.*, 2003) where all professions are assessed simultaneously. In this format, however, there is a tendency for students to distribute their scores across each row. In other words, a student might rate doctors 1 on their breadth of life experience, nurses a 2, social workers a 3, and so on. If these professions had been rated separately, then all professions may have potentially scored equally on this characteristic.
- develop alternative versions of the survey tool that are each distributed uniformly to the student cohort. For example, Hean *et al.* (2006a, 2006b) created four questionnaire versions, each asking for ratings of all characteristics but on a different subset of professions. The four versions were distributed proportionally across each professional group. Hereby data was collected on all characteristics on all professional groups. This reduced length of the questionnaire improved response rates. The main draw back of this approach, however, is that the sample size is effectively reduced four fold and is most suitable for evaluations using large student cohorts.

Table 8.3 Potential Format for Collecting Ratings on a Wide Range of Professional Groups (Carpenter *et al.*, 2003)

Indicate your views on the professions. Rate each profession on the following characteristics using a number between 1 (very low) and 7 (very high). A score of 4 = I don't know.

	Social workers	CPNs	OTs	Psychiatrists	Psychologists
Academic rigour	☐	☐	☐	☐	☐
Interpersonal skills (e.g. warmth, empathy)	☐	☐	☐	☐	☐

Content of questionnaire

Another practical challenge to stereotype measurement is the fact that students' responses to stereotype questions may be unduly influenced by what other questions appear in the same questionnaire tool.

Comparison of other professions being rated

First, if stereotypes of a doctor are assessed in the same questionnaire, in which stereotypes of mass murderers are rated, then doctors are likely to be assessed very favourably. This positive assessment of doctors may be less extreme, however, if nurses are the other group being rated in the questionnaire. Evaluators need, therefore, to be cogent of these contrasts students draw and the potential impact of this (Doosje *et al.*, 1998).

Inclusion and salience of professional identity

Second, it is argued elsewhere that professional identity is a covariate that should be considered alongside any measure of stereotype change (Hean and Dickinson, 2005; Hean and Macleod Clark, 2006; Hind *et al.*, 2003). If the mediating role of professional identity has not been taken into account, overall stereotype change (or the lack of it) may be misunderstood or misinterpreted. Practically, Cinnirella (1998) warns, however, that including identity questions in an evaluation tool alongside stereotype ratings may make professional identity more salient to students than it might be otherwise. This is likely to influence students' responses to both identity and stereotype questions.

Analysis

When stereotype ratings have been collected, evaluators will turn to means of analysis, whether this is to present baseline measures of existing stereotypes or to monitor change over time. Whilst a full discussion of statistical approaches is not appropriate here, it is worth drawing attention to the fact that evaluators take two views on analysis. In an analysis of the ratings given on individual characteristics (Boxes 8.2–8.5, Table 8.2 and Lindqvist *et al.*, 2005), some authors analyse the ratings of each stereotype characteristic independently (Carpenter, 1995b; Hean *et al.*, 2006a; Hean *et al.*, 2006b). Others have chosen to combine scores on each characteristic to form an overall stereotype score.

The latter assumes conceptually that ratings of stereotypical beliefs can be combined to form a measure of students' overall attitude. Hind *et al.* (2003) uses this approach, summing all ratings on each stereotype (reverse coding items were necessary). Similarly, Lindqvist *et al.* (2005) describe a two-factor underlying structure to the bipolar list of adjectives used: an overall *caring* and *subservient* dimension. The advantage of summing ratings on each characteristic is that the overall score may be conveniently used in correlations with other variables measured in an evaluation (e.g. with professional identity or readiness for interprofessional learning – Hind *et al.*, 2003). However, at a theoretical level, it may be argued that ratings on each individual characteristic are not sufficiently similar to represent an underlying construct called attitude to the professional group. It may also be questioned, whether each stereotype should receive an equal weighting, if the scores are to be summed, bearing in mind that different characteristics may be perceived as of more or less importance (Carpenter *et al.*, 2003).

At a more statistical level, the advisability of treating what is essentially ordinal data and non-additive data as continuous type data that can be manipulated in this way should also be assessed, as should the parametric/non-parametric nature of the data and the appropriateness of the statistical tests subsequently employed. The choice the evaluator makes will depend on the distribution of the data collected and the purity of the evaluators' statistical beliefs as to the extent a summation of a range of Likert, visual analogue or semantic differential items allows the data to approach continuous type measurement. The contentious argument that lies at the interface of statistics in the psychosocial sciences and the harder sciences is beyond the scope of this chapter.

Findings from studies using stereotypes as part of an evaluation

This chapter concludes by consideration of some of the results of studies in which stereotypes have been included.

HSC students do hold stereotypes of other professional groups

IPE evaluations have found that students do hold stereotypes of both their own and other professionals. These stereotypes exist at every educational level:

- In qualified professionals involved in career development IPE (Barnes *et al.*, 2000; Carpenter *et al.*, 2003);
- In final year students reaching the end of their pre-registration training (Carpenter, 1995b, 1995a; Carpenter and Hewstone, 1996);
- As early as at entry to their pre-registration training (Hind *et al.*, 2003; Tunstall-Pedoe *et al.*, 2003; Hean *et al.*, 2006a; Hean *et al.*, 2006b).

Students hold stereotypical views of other professional groups on a wide range of characteristics

Hean *et al.* (2006a), studying students on entry to a range of HSC pre-registration programmes, found that students saw midwives, social workers and nurses as high in interpersonal skills and being team players, and doctors as high in academic ability. Doctors, midwives and social workers were perceived as the strongest leaders and doctors were strong on decision-making. Similarly, medical and nursing students, in their final year of training, have been shown to stereotype nurses as caring, dedicated, good communicators, of greater breadth of life experience and doctors as confident, dedicated, arrogant and academically more able (Carpenter, 1995b). Medical and social work students (Hewstone *et al.*, 1994; Carpenter and Hewstone, 1996) stereotyped doctors as of higher academic ability and social workers as of greater breadth of life experience. Both groups were seen as professionally competent. Finally, in a career development programme of IPE for community mental health teams, similar stereotypes flourished with psychiatrists being rated highly as leaders. Social workers were not rated highly on this characteristic but were rated highly in terms of their interpersonal skills (Barnes *et al.*, 2000).

Similarity in profiles

Some evaluators choose to look at the stereotypes of each individual characteristic in parallel and develop an overall profile of the way in which a particular professional group is viewed. Instead of considering each characteristic of a profession in isolation, a stereotype profile is produced, in which all characteristics are plotted on the same axes, and the stereotypical strengths and weaknesses of the professional group compared (Hean *et al.*, 2006a). Scores are not summed but a visual representation of all ratings on all characteristics is presented instead (Figure 8.1; Hean *et al.*, 2006a).

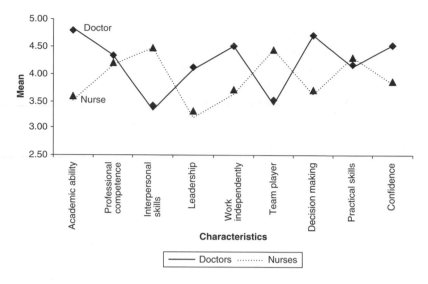

Figure 8.1 A comparison of the stereotype profiles of nurses and doctors (Hean *et al.*, 2006a)

In considering these profiles, Hean *et al.* (2006a) found that doctors and pharmacists were stereotyped in a similar fashion. Nurses, social workers and midwives also shared a similar profile. The profiles of nurses and doctors were perceived to be different. It is not yet known the impact that these similar stereotype profiles may have on inter-professional behaviour, whether similar profiles may stimulate feelings of empathy or whether very differently profiled professions may inter-act in a complementary or alternatively confrontational manner (Hean *et al.*, 2006a).

Lindqvist *et al.* (2005) also chose to consider the ratings of students on a series of characteristics heuristically, although they did so through the creation of two stereotype sub-scales discussed earlier. They found, similarly to Hean *et al.* (2006a), that pharmacists and doctors are char-acterised similarly on these broad constructs, both professional groups being low on the subservience and caring scales. Occupational thera-pists, nurses, physiotherapists and midwives are also viewed similarly being higher on both these dimensions.

Stereotype change

Stereotype change has been demonstrated during IPE programmes but results are inconclusive. An evaluation of IPE for medical, nursing

(Carpenter, 1995b) and social work students (Hewstone *et al.*, 1994; Carpenter and Hewstone, 1996) revealed an improvement in stereotypes in general over the programme. However, in subsequent evaluations of IPE with community health service workers, no statistically significant stereotype change was detected (Barnes *et al.*, 2000). In other cases, stereotypes may have become more negative (Tunstall-Pedoe *et al.*, 2003; Mandy *et al.*, 2004). These variations in findings arise potentially from some key conditions of contact being unmet (Barnes *et al.*, 2000). It may also occur if the curriculum being evaluated has not had stereotype change as an explicit learning outcome. Broadly speaking, stereotypes are known to be hard to change, having developed over an extensive period in the students' lives before they have even arrived for training. Positive stereotypes are particularly hard to develop (Rothbart and John, 1985) and it may take more than a single term (Tunstall-Pedoe *et al.*, 2003; Mandy *et al.*, 2004) of working together for these entrenched views to change.

Bearing in mind the above findings and that stereotypes are not a unidimensional construct, evaluators should be clear as to the type of stereotype change IPE might be expected to achieve. The following questions may help this process:

- Is it the nature of the stereotype that needs to be altered in students (e.g. Do we wish students to recognise the academic ability of all groups and rate all groups higher on this characteristic in the future)?
- Are we trying to foster mutual differentiation and a recognition that the professions have different strengths that are complementary in the HSC team?
- Does IPE develop reflective practitioners that through *knowledge* of the existing stereotypes. Their purpose and processes of meta-cognition, have the ability to identify their own intergroup behaviours?
- Are we trying to improve the value or importance placed on some characteristics, for example that being a team player is as important as being academically able?
- Is IPE trying to reduce the process of stereotyping itself through showing students that other professional groups are not homogeneous in their attributes?

These questions, especially the last three questions, remain largely inconclusive or unanswered in the IPE research.

Findings on mutual group differentiation

Applying social identity theory implied that good intergroup relations are promoted if students see their professional group as distinctive on certain characteristics, a fact optimised if this distinction is recognised by other professional groups (mutual intergroup differentiation). Hewstone *et al.* (1994) found that social work students saw themselves, and were seen by student doctors, as superior on life experience. Similarly, doctors saw themselves, and were seen by social workers, as superior on academic quality. Students therefore saw themselves as distinct and superior on particular characteristics and these same distinctions were recognised by other groups also.

In a similar evaluation, Carpenter (1995b) also found such consensus with '... nurses ... seen by both groups as caring, dedicated and good communicators and neither arrogant nor detached; doctors were confident, decisive and dedicated but arrogant' (Carpenter, 1995b:159). Barnes *et al.* (2000), in their evaluation of a post-registration IPE course, again found evidence of mutual intergroup differentiation in that 'social workers, community psychiatric nurses and occupational therapists were willing to concede superiority in leadership and academic rigor to psychiatrists and psychologists, but saw themselves as clearly superior in terms of communication, interpersonal and practical skills' (Barnes *et al.*, 2000:575).

Finally, Hean and Macleod Clark (2006) suggest that most first year HSC students perceived their professional ingroup as distinct from other professional groups, with the exception of audiology students. They conclude that the ability of students to see themselves as distinctive bodes well for future intergroup interactions. Furthermore, in certain groups there was evidence that student groups were seen by others, as they saw themselves. This was particularly the case for doctors and social workers and implies that these professions will suffer least from a threat to their group distinctiveness. However, there were instances where characteristics, seen as distinctive by the professional group itself, were not recognised by other groups. For example, physiotherapy students believe that being a team player, and decision-making and practical skills were all distinctive characteristics of their profession. However, these features were not recognised as distinctive by other professional groups. It is yet unknown how these matches/mismatches in how students see themselves, and how they may be viewed by others, impact on student learning experiences and relationships during IPE.

Conclusion

In this chapter, I have outlined some of the theoretical reasons for evaluating stereotype change in an IPE evaluation and summarised some of the measurements used to achieve this. There are some practical challenges and caveats, some of which may contribute to the variation in findings in this area. However, our understanding of stereotype change and the processes that underpin this is still underdeveloped. We need to explore the other dimensions of stereotype construct in greater detail. We need to better understand the impact of other variables on this construct, the influence of professional identity in particular, and we need to understand why stereotype change does not always occur. A structured assessment of the contact conditions in place during a programme has contributed to such an understanding (Barnes *et al.*, 2000) but this needs to be further developed. In addition, studies on stereotype change in IPE are also exclusively quantitative in nature. To explore this complex construct and the processes in IPE that underpin it, more qualitative approaches to measurement should be taken to triangulate with existing findings. Finally and perhaps most importantly, the relationship between stereotype ratings, stereotype change and any behavioural change at micro- and macro-levels of analysis are essential, if the evidence base supporting IPE and its potential impact is to be strengthened.

Acknowledgement

I would like to acknowledge the inputs of Professor Alex Haslam (University of Exeter) and Professor John Carpenter (University of Bristol) to my understanding of this area and the content of this chapter.

References

Allport, G.W. (1979). *The Nature of Prejudice*. Cambridge, MA: Perseus Books Publishing, L.L.C.

Barnes, D., J. Carpenter and C. Dickinson. (2000). Interprofessional education for community mental health: Attitudes to community care and professional stereotypes. *Social Work Education*, 565–583.

Barnes, D., J. Carpenter and C. Dickinson. (2006). The outcomes of partnerships with mental health service users in interprofessional education: A case study. *Health & Social Care in the Community*, 14(5), 426–435.

Branscombe, N.R., N. Ellemers, R. Spears and B. Doosje. (1999). The context and content of social identity threat. In N. Ellemers, R. Spears and B. Doosje (eds), *Social Identity, Context, Commitment, Content*. Oxford: Blackwell Publishers.

Brown, R., S. Condor, A. Matthews and G. Wade. (1986). Explaining intergroup differentiation in an industrial organization. *Journal of Occupational Psychology*, 59(4), 273–286.

Carpenter, J. (1995a). Doctors and nurses: Stereotypes and stereotype change in interprofessional education. *Journal of Interprofessional Care*, 9(2), 151–161.

Carpenter, J. (1995b). Interprofessional education for medical and nursing students: Evaluation of a programme. *Medical Education*, 29(4), 265–272.

Carpenter, J. and M. Hewstone. (1996). Shared learning for doctors and social workers: Evaluation of a programme. *British Journal of Social Work*, 26(2), 239–257.

Carpenter, J., D. Barnes and C. Dickinson. (2003). *Making a Modern Mental Health Care Workforce: Evaluation of the Birmingham University Interprofessional Training Programme in Community Mental Health 1998–2002*. Durham: Centre for Applied Social Studies, University of Durham.

Cinnirella, M. (1998). Manipulating stereotype rating tasks: Understanding questionnaire context effects on measures of attitudes, social identity and stereotypes. *Journal of Community & Applied Social Psychology*, 8(5), 345–362.

Conroy, R.M., M. Teehan, R. Siriwardena, O. Smyth, H.M. McGee and P. Fernandes. (2002). Attitudes to doctors and medicine: The effect of setting and doctor-patient relationship. *British Journal of Health Psychology*, 7(1), 117–125.

Doosje, B., S.A. Haslam, R. Spears, P.J. Oakes, and W. Koomen. (1998). The effect of comparative context on central tendency and variability judgements and the evaluation of group characteristics. *European Journal of Social Psychology*, 28(2), 173–184.

Du Toit, D. (1995). A sociological analysis of the extent and influence of professional socialization on the development of a nursing identity among nursing students at two universities in Brisbane, Australia. *Journal of Advanced Nursing*, 21(1), 164–171.

Fishbein, M. and I. Ajzen. (1975). *Belief, Attitude, Intention and Behaviour – An Introduction to Theory and Behaviour*. Reading, MA: Addison-Wesley Publishing Company.

Freeth, D., M. Hammick, I. Koppel, S. Reeves and H. Barr. (2002). *A Critical Review of Evaluations of Interprofessional Education*. London: LTSN-Centre for Health Sciences and Practices.

Hallam, J. (2000). *Nursing the Image: Media, Culture and Professional Identity*. London: Routledge.

Haslam, S.A., C. Powell and J.C.Turner. (2000). Social identity, self-categorization, and work motivation: Rethinking the contribution of the group to positive and sustainable organisational outcomes. *Applied Psychology: An International Review*, 49(3), 319.

Haslam, S.A., J.C. Turner, P.J. Oakes, J.K. Reynolds, B. Doosje, C. McGarty, *et al.* (2002). *From Personal Pictures in the Head to Collective Tools in the World: How Shared Stereotypes Allow Groups to Represent and Change Social Reality*. New York, US: Cambridge University Press.

Hean, S., J. Macleod Clark, D. Humphris and K. Adams. (2003). *Can Stereotypes Be Measured? Conference in Interprofessional Learning in Health and Social Care.* London: Association for Medical Education (ASME).

Hean, S. and C. Dickinson. (2005). The contact hypothesis: An exploration of its further potential in interprofessional education. *Journal of Interprofessional Care,* 19(5), 480–491.

Hean, S. and J. Macleod Clark. (2006). Poster presentation: Them against us? Group identity & students' perceptions of other health & social care professional groups, Altogether Better Health III. London.

Hean, S., J. Macleod Clark, K. Adams and D. Humphris. (2006a). Will opposites attract? Similarities and differences in students' perceptions of the stereotype profiles of other health and social care professional groups. *Journal of Interprofessional Care,* 20(2), 162–181.

Hean, S., J. Macleod Clark, K. Adams, D. Humphris and J. Lathlean. (2006b). Being seen by others as we see ourselves: Ingroup and outgroup perceptions of health and social care students. *Learning in Health and Social Care,* 5, 10–22.

Hewstone, M. and R. Brown. (1986). *Contact Is not Enough: An Intergroup Perspective on the 'Contact Hypothesis'.* Cambridge, MA, US: Basil Blackwell.

Hewstone, M., J. Carpenter, A. Franklyn-Stokes and D. Routh (1994). Intergroup contact between professional groups: Two evaluation studies. *Journal of Community & Applied Social Psychology,* 4(5), 347–363.

Hewstone, M. and J. Hamberger. (2000). Perceived variability and stereotype change. *Journal of Experimental Social Psychology,* 36(2), 103–124.

Hilton, J.L. and W. Von Hippel. (1996). Stereotypes. *Annual Review of Psychology,* 47, 237–271.

Hind, M., I. Norman, S. Cooper, E. Gill, R. Hilton, P. Judd, *et al.* (2003). Interprofessional perceptions of health care students. *Journal of Interprofessional Care,* 17(1), 21–34.

Kirkham, M., H. Stapleton, P. Curtis and G. Thomas. (2002). Stereotyping as a professional defence mechanism. (Cover story). *British Journal of Midwifery,* 10(9), 549.

Kirkpatrick, D.L. (1967). *Evaluation of Training.* New York: McGraw-Hill.

Leaviss, J. (2000). Exploring the perceived effect of an undergraduate multiprofessional educational intervention. *Medical Education,* 34(6), 483–486.

Lindqvist, S., A. Duncan, L. Shepstone, F. Watts and S. Pearce. (2005). Development of the 'Attitudes to Health Professionals Questionnaire' (AHPQ): A measure to assess interprofessional attitudes. *Journal of Interprofessional Care,* 19(3), 269–279.

Mandy, A., C. Milton and P. Mandy. (2004). Professional stereotyping and interprofessional education. *Learning in Health and Social Care,* 3, 154–170.

O'Halloran, C., S. Hean, D. Humphris and J. Macleod-Clark. (2006). Developing common learning: The new generation project undergraduate curriculum model. *Journal of Interprofessional Care,* 20(1), 12–28.

Pettigrew, T.F. (1997). Generalized intergroup contact effects on prejudice. *Personality and Social Psychology Bulletin,* 23, 173–185.

Rothbart, M. and O.P. John. (1995). Social categorization and behavioural episode: A cognitive analysis of the effects of intergroup contact. *Journal of Social Issues,* 41, 81–104.

Stephan, W.G. and C.W. Stephan. (1984). The role of ignorance in intergroup relations. In N. Miller and M.B. Brewer (Eds), *Groups in Contact*. New York: Academic Press.

Tajfel, H., M.G. Billig, R.P. Bundy and C. Flament. (1971). Social categorization and intergroup behaviour. *European Journal of Social Psychology*, 1, 149–178.

Takase, M., E. Kershaw and L. Burt. (2002). Does public image of nurses matter? *Journal of Professional Nursing*, 18(4), 196–205.

Tunstall-Pedoe, S., E. Rink and S. Hilton. (2003). Student attitudes to undergraduate interprofessional education. *Journal of Interprofessional Care*, 17(2), 161–172.

Turner, J.C. (1999). Some current issues in research on social identity and self categorization theories. In N. Ellemers, R. Spears and B. Doosje (eds), *Social Identity, Context, Commitment, Content* (pp. 6–34). Oxford: Blackwell Publishers.

Zárate, M.A. and A.A. Garza. (2002). In-group distinctiveness and self-affirmation as dual components of prejudice reduction. *Self and Identity*, 1(3), 235–249.

9

The 'Attitudes to Health Professionals Questionnaire' (AHPQ)

Suzanne Lindqvist

Introduction

Background

I work together with my colleagues in the Centre for Interprofessional Practice at the University of East Anglia (UEA), Norwich, UK. The Centre was founded in 2002 with the aim of developing an interprofessional learning (IPL) programme. At the outset of the planning of the IPL programme, we discussed ways in which we could evaluate its effectiveness. The aim of the IPL programme is for participants to develop the knowledge, skills, attitudes and behaviour that facilitate effective interprofessional teamworking. Our interest focuses in particular on the development of positive interprofessional attitudes, as we feel this plays a pivotal role in the communication and interaction amongst healthcare professionals.

Views about what it is like working together with different healthcare professionals emerge long before the end of professional training (McPherson *et al.* 2001). Indeed, students have been shown to enter their healthcare training with views about their own professional role, and the role of others (Carpenter 1995; Tunstall-Pedoe *et al.* 2003; Lindqvist *et al.* 2005). Furthermore, differences in how professions are perceived exist in clinical settings (Mackay 1993; Walby *et al.* 1994). Should these views translate into negative attitudes, they may inhibit communication between different healthcare professionals (Areskog 1988; Mackay 1993; Parsell *et al.* 1998), which can have an undesirable effect on patient care (Ryan and McKenna 1994).

With this in mind, we started to look at the wider literature to see what already existed in terms of validated tools that could be used to measure interprofessional attitudes. The Interdisciplinary Education Perception Scale (IEPS) developed by Luecht and colleagues (1990) is a validated scale designed to assess students' views of their own profession in relation to others. However, the IEPS cannot be used to measure students' views of a range of *different* healthcare professions. Neither does it focus on personal attributes, but rather issues associated directly with interprofessional teamworking. This is also the case with the Readiness for Interprofessional Learning Scale (RIPLS), developed by Parsell and Bligh (1999) with the aim of measuring students' attitudes and willingness to engage in interprofessional education (IPE).

Carpenter (1995) described a 'Health Care Stereotype Scale', which can be used to measure interprofessional attitudes. However, this scale looks only at a limited number of personal descriptors and was not validated in a setting that included a number of different healthcare professionals.

As we could not find a validated tool, suitable for what we had set out to measure, we decided to develop an instrument that could be used for our own purposes and interest, and that was applicable to a *range* of healthcare professionals. We named the tool the Attitudes to Health Professionals Questionnaire (AHPQ). This chapter will briefly describe the process in which the AHPQ was developed and validated, and the way it has been used over the past four years. The method of analysis, applied by the people involved in the development, will be explained and comments will be made on the strengths and weaknesses of this tool. Some findings from using the AHPQ will be shared, both in relation to its use internally, and also when comparing findings of other sites when using this measure. Hopefully, this will provide an overview of how this tool can be applied.

Process of development

The AHPQ was developed with the aim of understanding differences in attitudes between healthcare professional groups, and evaluation of attitudinal change over time. The term 'attitudes' in the title of this measure is defined as an indicator of how people make sense of their experience (Eiser 1997). The development of this questionnaire will be briefly described below and for further details see the full article by myself and colleagues in 2005 (Lindqvist *et al.* 2005).

The development took place in two stages.

Stage one

The questionnaire contains 20 items, and each item consists of two opposite attributes. The 20 items were elicited from staff members across the health schools at UEA, by asking them to consider three professions and then to describe how two of these were seen as similar, but different to the third. This way of extracting personal constructs originates from a method described by Kelly (1955). A 10 cm visual analogue scale was used, and each part of the item served as verbal anchors for each end of the scale.

For example, flexible/not flexible:

Flexible   Not flexible

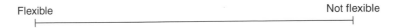

One hundred and ninety students from five different professions in the academic year 2002–2003 agreed to be part of the development of the questionnaire by completing it on two occasions. The students were asked to rate each item in relation to a typical member of a certain profession by putting a cross on the visual analogue scale.

The AHPQ is divided into a number of sections, with the same 20 items in each section, and each section representing a different healthcare profession. The number of sections, and thus the length, of the AHPQ is therefore dependent upon the number of healthcare professions included. In our IPL programme, a student will answer 20 items referring to their own profession, and then will give answers to the same items for each one of the other healthcare professions that were part of their IPL group. Generally, an IPL group consists of—six to eight students from at least four different professions. For the development and validation of the AHPQ, students completed five sections. Nowadays students will only complete four sections to make it a less onerous task.

Data collated from 190 students were analysed using SPSS version 11. To assess its internal structure and reliability, they were subjected to the following tests:

- Principal components analysis;
- Cronbach's alpha coefficient;
- Individual test–retest intra-class correlation coefficient (ICC).

Principal components analysis

The principal components analysis involves a mathematical procedure that groups the 20 items into a reduced number of uncorrelated variables called *principal components*. The main principal component accounts for as much of the variability in the data as possible, and each succeeding component accounts for the remaining variability (Bryman and Cramer 1997). The number of students included was considered appropriate for exploratory principal components analysis (Oppenheim 1992).

Two main components, which we labelled 'caring' and 'subservient', emerged from the principal components analysis accounting for 43% of the total variance, and with 17 of the 20 items loading on these 2 components.

Cronbach's alpha coefficient

The Cronbach's alpha gives an indication of the internal consistency of items, and thus to what extent the items are correlated with each other. The alpha coefficient ranges between 0 (no consistency) and 1 (total consistency), with values greater than 0.7 being deemed as reliable (McKinley *et al.* 1997).

The internal consistency for the original 20-item questionnaire was high ($\alpha > 0.86$). The alpha coefficients were also calculated for each component to assess the respective reliability. The 'caring' component was the strongest, and accounted for 33% of the total variance. Thirteen items loaded on this component, which showed good internal consistency ($\alpha > 0.91$). The 'subservient' component accounted for 10% of the total variance and the items loading on this component had an internal consistency of 0.59.

Individual test–retest intra-class correlation coefficient

The test–retest protocol demonstrates how rigorous a questionnaire is in terms of how reproducible the data are when measuring the same subject twice. By calculating ICCs on these data we could assess how reliable the data obtained from the questionnaire were. Here, 1 represents perfect agreement between tests, whereas 0 represents no agreement at all, with values greater than 0.9 indicating a high reliability and reproducibility of the questionnaire.

Test–retest ICC was calculated for each item and was shown to vary between 0.34 and 0.85. According to Nunnally (1978), test–retest measures are considered adequately high if equal to or greater than 0.7.

After subjecting the data collated from the initial questionnaire to these tests, some items were considered for removal or rephrasing, leading us on to stage two of the development.

Stage two

The initial questionnaire was revised in the light of the data emerging from the statistical test, with some of the items removed or changed if the:

- principal component loading was less than 0.5;
- Cronbach's alpha coefficient increased when an item was removed;
- test–retest ICC was less than 0.7;
- anchors conflated two different constructs.

For detailed information about how the questionnaire was revised, please see the full article in Lindqvist *et al.* (2005).

Reassessment of the structure and reliability of the revised AHPQ

The same statistical tests were carried out on the revised questionnaire. As with the initial questionnaire, the 'caring' and 'subservient' components emerged from principal components analysis accounting for 50% of the total variance. The principal components scores are shown in Table 9.1.

Table 9.1   Principal Components Scores for the 'Caring' and 'Subservient' Scales

Item	Principal component (PC) score	
	PC 1 'caring' scale	PC 2 'subservient' scale
1. Technically focussed/not technically focussed	0.192	0.544
2. Values autonomy/does not value autonomy	–	.
3. Not patient-centred/patient-centred	0.755	−0.164
4. Assertive/non-assertive	−0.226	0.616
5. Arrogant/not arrogant	0.587	0.167
6. Not conciliatory/conciliatory	0.533	–
7. Well paid/poorly paid	0.488	0.490
8. Not thoughtful/thoughtful	0.792	−0.223
9. Theoretical/practical	0.545	0.219
10. Self-centred/not self-centred	0.733	–
11. Confident/vulnerable	−0.265	0.644
12. Non-sympathetic/sympathetic	0.816	–
13. Flexible/not flexible	0.791	–
14. Does not value team work/values teamwork	0.823	–
15. Confrontational/not confrontational	0.225	0.319

Table 9.1 Continued

Item	Principal component (PC) score	
	PC 1 'caring' scale	PC 2 'subservient' scale
16. Independent/not independent	0.131	0.521
17. Non-caring/caring	0.872	–
18. Non-empathetic/empathetic	0.839	–
19. Non-approachable/approachable	0.833	–
20. Rough/gentle	0.673	–

Note: Items in bold have been randomly selected to be swapped around in the questionnaire. Please see below for further information.

For each paired item as shown in Table 9.1, the word/phrase on the left is considered 'cold' and the word/phrase on the right, 'warm'. These labels were confirmed through the correlation matrix during the principal components analysis. If a pair was the other way round, this was clear on the matrix and no correlation found. The internal consistency increased ($\alpha > 0.87$) for the 20-item questionnaire, and for the 'caring' and 'subservient' components, the alpha co-efficients were calculated at 0.93 and 0.58, respectively.

Following revision, the AHPQ was administered, at the outset of an IPL programme in 2003, to a new group of first year students ($n = 160$) from 6 different healthcare professions. This served as a primary validation of the questionnaire and the next section will explain how we analysed our data.

Data Analysis

Preparation and suggested protocol

When these data were analysed we used the paper version of the AHPQ. Now we have developed and use an online version of the questionnaire. There are differences in the preparation required for both the paper and the online questionnaires. This is because routine processes can be completed automatically with the online AHPQ. These same processes need to be completed by hand with the paper AHPQ and are described below. In general, the online AHPQ is ready for data analysis and you could proceed directly to the section 'calculating principal component scores'.

Table 9.2 Suggested Data Input Style for Excel/SPSS, Showing 9 of the 20 Columns

	Fi1	Fi2	Fi3	Fi4	Fi5	Fi6	Fi7	Fi8	Fi9
Student 1	3.3	2.2	9.3	7.3	4.9	2.6	9.7	3.3	8.7
Student 2	4.2	1.6	8.6	8.4	5.3	3.1	8.2	3.4	7.4

Notes: F = administration of the AHPQ first time around; i = label for 'pharmacist'; 1–9 = represents the items (so should be columns up to 20).

Preparing raw data

Before you start, always remember to keep a record of the raw data. When calculating a principal component score for each student for the two scales, only completed data can be used. This means that for every student, there needs to be a score for each of the 20 items on the scale. Each student's score needs to be measured and entered into Excel or SPSS manually. For the purposes of storing raw data and subsequent data analysis we have assumed the following input style (Table 9.2):

We have implemented the following shortened labels:

> We differentiate between when the questionnaire was administered: first time (F) or second time (S). For example, if the questionnaire is distributed prior to an IPL programme, the answers would have an 'F' as a label and the second distribution would be after the programme (S).

> We label for each section of the AHPQ corresponding to the different healthcare professionals representing each section. Some examples are:

> > i = Pharmacist
> > ii = Occupational Therapist
> > iii = Medic

Finally, we use the relevant item number e.g. 1, 2 or 3, etc.

To summarise, and give some examples, the data labels would be as follows:

Fi1 = first time around, pharmacist, item 1
Fi2 = first time around, pharmacist, item 2

Fii1 = first time around, occupational therapist, item 1
Sii1 = second time around, occupational therapist, item 1
Siii12 = second time around, medic, item 12

In order to carry out statistical tests on the data collected from the AHPQ, the following three steps need to be completed:

- Filling in missing data;
- Swapping items around;
- Calculating principal component scores.

Filling in missing data

The missing data need to be dealt with prior to data analysis, by either withdrawing or calculating an average on incomplete data sets. This needs to be done only when using the paper questionnaire, as this function is built-in when using the online version.

Swapping items around

This is also the case when considering the way in which 'warm' and 'cold' attributes are presented in an item. We have mixed the orientation of the attributes in items, so that a 'cold' word/phrase is not always arranged on the left and 'warm' on the right. This will help ensure students are considering each item individually when scoring. However, in order for us to carry out principal components analysis on the data, these items need to be swapped around so that the 'cold' concepts are given the correct scores.

For the paper questionnaire, we use an Excel spreadsheet, transferring the raw data to a new spreadsheet and then using a formula to recalculate the score. The swapped data can then be transferred into SPSS ready for analysis. Table 9.1 shows the items where data needs to be swapped around (so if a score of 3.5 has been given for item 3, knowing that the visual analogue scale is 10 cm, the data point needs to be 'corrected' to 6.5 as it was swapped around for the purpose of the questionnaire).

Calculating principal component scores

For the 'caring' and 'subservient' scales, each item has a different weighting on the scale. These are the same as shown in Table 9.1. In order to analyse the data using the two different scales ('caring' and 'subservient'), a series of calculations will turn the data into a series of scores for each student and for each scale. This calculation can be done by typing in the label for the relevant item and multiplying it by the weighting on the scale. However, to make it an easier process, we designed a formula for this, which could be copied into the calculation, reducing laborious work and the possibility of error.

For the purpose of the formulae and the limitations of SPSS, we gave each score a label. To give some examples, the data labels would be as follows:

For Component 1, asking about a typical pharmacist first time around: C1PH1

For Component 1, asking about a typical pharmacist second time around: C1PH2

For Component 2, asking about a typical medic first time around: C2ME1

For Component 2, asking about a typical medic second time around: C2ME2

To calculate the principal component scores in SPSS go to: 'transform' and click 'compute'. When prompted, add in the 'target variable name' and paste in the formula shown in Table 9.3.

In SPSS head columns by the target variable name used in each case. Table 9.4 shows you how.

By carrying out this procedure in SPSS, the scores will be automatically added into the appropriate column. It is these principal component scores that are later used for any data representation, or further statistical analysis.

Statistical analysis

Apart from calculating the means and standard deviations to summarise the key features of the data, we have used paired samples t-test and analysis of variance (ANOVA) to test whether there are any significant differences within groups and between groups.

Paired samples t-test

Having calculated the principal component scores for each profession, and for each of the two scales, we used this test to see whether students' views at the beginning of the IPL programme were different from those measured at the end. The paired samples t-test will test whether the means of each student score differ.

Table 9.3 Formulae for Calculating Principal Component Scores

Component 1 – 'Caring' Scale

Target variable	Formula
C1PH1	Fi1 * .192 + Fi3 * .755 + Fi4 * −.226 + Fi5 * .587 + Fi6 * .533 + Fi7 * .488 + Fi8 * .792 + Fi9 * .545 + Fi10 * .733 + Fi11 * −.265 + Fi12 * .816 + Fi13 * .791 + Fi14 * .823 + Fi15 * .225 + Fi16 * .131 + Fi17 * .872 + Fi18 * .839 + Fi19 * .833 + Fi20 * .673
C1PH2	Si1 * .192 + Si3 * .755 + Si4 * −.226 + Si5 * .587 + Si6 * .533 + Si7 * .488 + Si8 * .792 + Si9 * .545 + Si10 * .733 + Si11 * −.265 + Si12 * .816 + Si13 * .791 + Si14 * .823 + Si15 * .225 + Si16 * .131 + Si17 * .872 + Si18 * .839 + Si19 * .833 + Si20 * .673

Component 2 – 'Subservient' scale

C2ME1	Fiii1 * .544 + Fiii2 * .554 + Fiii3 * −.164 + Fiii4 * .616 + Fiii5 * .167 + Fiii7 * .490 + Fiii8 * −.223 + Fiii9 * .219 + Fiii11 * .644 + Fiii15 * .319 + Fiii16 * .521
C2ME2	Siii1 * .544 + Siii2 * .554 + Siii3 * −.164 + Siii4 * .616 + Siii5 * .167 + Siii7 * .490 + Siii8 * −.223 + Siii9 * .219 + Siii11 * .644 + Siii15 * .319 + Siii16 * .521

Table 9.4 Data Input in SPSS

	C1PH1	C1PH2	C1OT1	C1OT2	C1ME1	C1ME2
Student 1						
Student 2						

In SPSS go to 'analyse' and 'compare means' choosing 'paired samples *t*-test'. Select which two variables you would like to compare, for example C1PH1 and C1PH2. This will test the means of all student scores for Component 1 (the 'caring' scale) and thus the students' views of a typical pharmacist before and after they have worked together in an IPL group.

ANOVA

This test enables analysis between the calculated means from three or more different professions, which cannot be done with a *t*-test.

The ANOVA tells us whether the means of students' perceptions of nurses, medics and pharmacists for Component 1 first time around are similar. A significant value indicates that at least one group (profession) is different, but it does not tell you which one. A separate ANOVA would need to be carried out on data collated from each profession the second time students completed the AHPQ (i.e. after the IPL programme).

To carry out the procedure, in SPSS go to 'analyse', 'compare means' selecting the appropriate ANOVA, and choose which professions you wish to compare.

Findings from the Questionnaire

Primary validation of the revised questionnaire

Figure 9.1 shows results of the data collated from 160 students, included in the preliminary validation of the revised questionnaire. In brief, these results show that there are clear differences in students' views towards healthcare professionals at the outset of the IPL programme. Differences

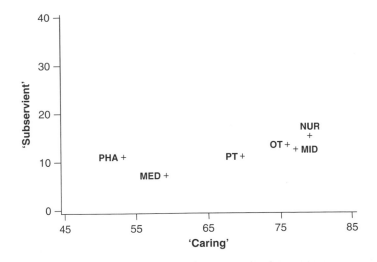

Figure 9.1 Plot of mean scores on both the 'caring' and 'subservient' axes showing differences in students' attitudes towards each profession at the outset of their training (Lindqvist *et al.* 2005)

in both mean 'caring' and 'subservient' scores were observed, some of which were significant. Students viewed a typical pharmacist as being the least 'caring' professional and the typical nurse as being the most 'caring' professional. Nurses were seen as significantly more 'subservient' than doctors. For further details please see the full article in Lindqvist *et al.* (2005).

These preliminary data were later confirmed by including a new group of students, and these data also detected changes over time.

Further Validation of the AHPQ

A new group of 179 first year students from 6 different healthcare professions, in the academic year of 2003/2004, completed the questionnaire at the outset, and at the end of the IPL programme. As illustrated in Figure 9.2, these results confirmed the preliminary findings presented in Figure 9.1.

Since presenting findings obtained from this questionnaire, other sites have become interested in using this tool. One site is Holstebro Hospital in Denmark, with whom we have initiated collaboration.

AHPQ data collated and analysed in a different setting

The Interprofessional Training Unit (ITU) at Holstebro Hospital initiated a three year project in the Clinic of Orthopaedics in 2004. The ITU is a collaborative project between Central Denmark Region, the Schools of Occupational Therapy, Physiotherapy and Nursing and the Faculty of Health Sciences at the University of Aarhus. Together, with staff at ITU, we converted the AHPQ, by first translating each item into Danish, then translating them back into English, each process being carried out by two independent people, and then finally agreeing on a final version of a Danish questionnaire via a telephone conference. This process of translation was inspired by work from Beaton and colleagues (2000).

Students from ITU (including occupational therapists, physiotherapists, nurses and doctors) have since completed a Danish version of the AHPQ. Data, similar to those presented by us, have been presented by Flemming Jacobsen, both nationally and internationally. In his research, each of the professional groups were viewed by students as being more 'caring' after a two-week stay in the ITU, with the greatest difference

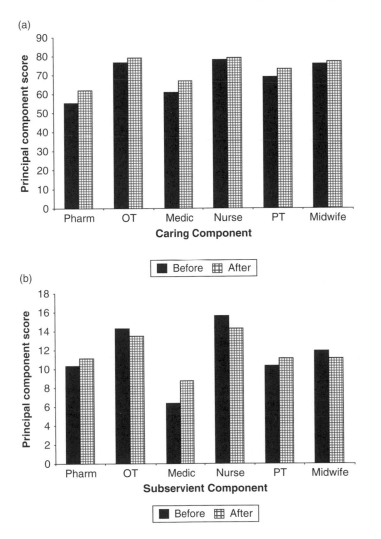

Figure 9.2 Bar charts showing mean scores before and after the IPL programme for the (a) 'caring' and (b) 'subservient' components, respectively

observed in the students' views of doctors, followed by their views of occupational therapists, then physiotherapists, with the smallest difference being in their views of nurses. Only small changes were seen on the 'subservient' component. The Danish version of the AHPQ will be revalidated in this new setting and quantitative data will be supported with qualitative data.

Other sites have also started using the AHPQ to help evaluate the impact on their IPL initiatives and on interprofessional attitudes. Hopefully, these data will help contribute to our understanding of this complex area, and also provide interesting information about social aspects of the development of such attitudes, and how we can best influence them in a positive manner.

Strengths and Weaknesses

We have found this questionnaire very helpful, as it has confirmed to us, and the students themselves, that students have different views of their own and other healthcare professions and that these attitudes change over time. The importance of this finding is yet to be determined and, like our colleagues in Denmark, we carry out interviews with students, in order to understand interprofessional attitudes in more depth, their impact on interprofessional working in practice, and how we can optimise opportunities for IPL to promote the development of positive attitudes.

Validation of the questionnaire shows good internal consistency and acceptable test–retest reliability. The 'caring' component is strong, whereas the 'subservient' component is weaker, accounting for less of a variance with lower reliability. However, further development of the questionnaire will be carried out, both in the pre- and post-registration setting. This is because more professional groups have joined the programme and thus more students and staff from whom we would like to elicit attributes to ensure the 20 items are still appropriate. Also, we would like to validate the AHPQ in the practice setting and include patients as we extend our post-registration IPL programme (Watts *et al.* 2007).

Access and more information about the questionnaire

We tend to give our students access to the online version of the AHPQ, as this is collecting the data and helps with the first steps of analysis, as described earlier. Should you be interested in viewing either the online

version or the paper version of the questionnaire please contact us at
http://www.uea.ac.uk/cipp/

Conclusion

There is still a call for more rigorous evidence to show the impact of
IPL on healthcare students' professional development and team performance. We need this evidence, if nothing else, to convince the
sceptics that the current investment in this – quite labour-intensive –
learning is worthwhile in terms of its long-lasting effect on improved
interprofessional practice and patient care.

Through developing and validating tools that can be used for this purpose, we can address this issue. The AHPQ is a questionnaire that can be
used to assess interprofessional attitudes. Attitudes in this context relate
to how a typical member of a profession is associated with a particular
attribute (e.g. approachable, assertive, thoughtful, patient-centred). The
AHPQ was developed for the purpose of understanding how healthcare
professionals view members of their own profession and those of other
professional groups. The questionnaire can be used to measure existing
attitudes and changes in attitudes over time, and as part of the evaluation of interventions such as students being part of IPL. The AHPQ has
been used for a number of years now showing reliable results in different
settings. Interesting findings have been presented here showing differences in students' views at the outset of their IPL experience, and that
these views had changed when measured after students have worked
together.

This chapter was written for those interested in using a validated tool
as a means to assess attitudes, for those who wanted to know more about
how it was developed, and more importantly, for those who wanted
some help with how to analyse the data collated from it. Needless to
say, the AHPQ needs to be complemented with other research methods
in order to fully understand interprofessional attitudes and their relation
to team performance and patient care.

References

Areskog, N-H. (1988).The need for multi-professional health education in undergraduate studies. *Medical Education* 22, 251–252.
Beaton, D.E., C. Bombardier, F. Guillemin and M.B. Ferraz. (2000). Guidelines for
the process of cross-cultural adaptation of self-report measures. *Spine* 25 (24), 6.

Bryman, A. and D. Cramer. (1997). *Quantitative Data Analysis with SPSS for Windows*. London: Routledge.

Carpenter, J. (1995). Doctors and nurses: Stereotypes and stereotype change in interprofessional education. *Journal of Interprofessional Care* 9 (2), 151–161.

Eiser, J.R. (1997). Attitudes and beliefs. In Baum, A., Newman, S., Weinmann, J., West, R. and McManns, C. (eds), *Cambridge Handbook of Psychology, Health and Medicine*. Cambridge: Cambridge University Press.

Kelly, G.A. (1955). *The Psychology of Personal Constructs*. New York: Norton.

Luecht, R.M., M.K. Madsen, M.P. Taugher and B.J. Petterson. (1990). Assessing professional perceptions: Design and validation of an interdisciplinary education perception scale. *Journal of Allied Health* 19 (2), 181–191.

Lindqvist, S., A. Duncan, L. Shepstone, F. Watts and S. Pearce. (2005). Development of the 'Attitudes to Health Professionals Questionnaire' (AHPQ): A measure to assess interprofessional attitudes. *Journal of Interprofessional Care* 19 (3), 269–279.

Mackay, L. (1993). *Conflicts in Care, Medicine and Nursing*. London: Chapman & Hall.

McKinley, R.K., T. Manku-Scott, A.M. Hastings, D.P. French and R. Baker. (1997). Reliability and validity of a new measure of patient satisfaction with out of hours primary medical care in the United Kingdom: Development of a patient questionnaire. *British Medical Journal* 314, 193–198.

McPherson, K., L. Headrick and F. Moss. (2001). Working and learning together; good quality care depends on it, but how do we achieve it? *Quality in Health Care* 10 (2), 46–53.

Nunnally, J.C. (1978). *Psychometric theory*, 2nd edition. New York: McGraw-Hill.

Oppenheim, A.N. (1992). *Questionnaire Design, Interviewing and Attitude Measurement*. London: Pinter Publishers.

Parsell, G., R. Spalding and J. Bligh. (1998). Shared goals, shared learning: Evaluation of a multi-professional course for undergraduate students. *Medical Education* 32, 304–311.

Parsell, G. and J. Bligh. (1999). The development of a questionnaire to assess the readiness of health care students for interprofessional learning (RIPLS). *Medical Education* 33, 95–100.

Ryan, A. and H. McKenna. (1994). A comparative study of the attitudes of nursing and medical students to aspects of patient care and the nurse's role in organizing that care. *Journal of Advanced Nursing* 19, 114–123.

Tunstall-Pedoe, S., E. Rink and S. Hilton. (2003). Student attitudes to undergraduate interprofessional education. *Journal of Interprofessional Care* 7 (2), 161–172.

Walby, S., J. Greenwell, L. Mackay and K. Soothill. (1994). *Medicine and Nursing: Professions in a Changing Health Service*. London: Sage.

Watts, F., S. Lindqvist, S. Pearce, M. de Lourdes Drachler and B. Richardson. (2007). Introducing an interprofessional learning programme for healthcare teams. *Medical Teacher* 29 (5), 457–463.

Part IV
Sustainability

This final part of the book consists of two chapters considering the challenges to sustaining interprofessional learning in education and practice. In Chapter 10 Ann Jackson and Patricia Bluteau draw on UK and international examples to demonstrate evidence of these challenges and move to propose a model which the authors consider is an essential element of interprofessional working and also for interprofessional education sustainability both within practice and academe. The chapter provides tips and guidance on managing change in both settings and builds on the models of IPE discussed in Part II of the book. In Chapter 11, the final chapter, Marilyn Hammick and Liz Anderson focus on sustainability in IPE by highlighting and drawing on models of IPE which have been developed and embedded in curricula and practice and as such have demonstrated that they are sustainable. Key messages are outlined in terms of human resources, developing effective local partnerships and using research and evaluation linked to a 'continuous quality cycle' which will help develop a sustainable approach to IPE.

David Guile.

10

Creating a Model: Overcoming the Challenges of Implementing Interprofessional Education

Ann Jackson and Patricia Bluteau

Introduction

The previous chapters in this book have considered the background issues in the development of interprofessional education (IPE) and explored the methods and settings for delivery. This chapter proposes a model of collaboration which includes a set of key components, considered essential to the creation of sustainable and successful IPE opportunities which will result in a flexible workforce (Chapter 2). The model is informed by the challenges and issues related to implementing IPE in both practice and academic settings.

This chapter breaks down the collaboration model by describing the requisite parts, whilst linking the challenges of delivering IPE within both face-to-face and virtual models of delivery. It will further unpack the underlying prerequisites which appear to be essential, yet which can often remain elusive, if IPE opportunities are to be sustainable and collaboration is to be achieved. In addition, this chapter will also address the covert issues that can act as barriers to the development of the interprofessional agenda.

A growing body of papers highlights the challenges to the delivery and implementation of IPE (Barker *et al.* 2005; Gilbert 2005; Jackson and Bluteau 2007), with most identifying the same difficulties which clearly focus on a range of themes that are widely experienced. Major barriers centre on the use of language, definition of IPE, impact of any change on profession and organisations, economic and resource barriers and the sheer logistics of implementing an activity across many different social and healthcare professional groups who have different curricula, timetables, length and educational requirements. Enablers to IPE centre on identification of champions and external support and resources. If we are to provide sustainable IPE to future generations of health and social care professions then we have to work to remove these barriers.

Revisiting the CAIPE Definition of IPE

It is important at this point to return to the Centre for Advancement of Interprofessional Education (CAIPE) definition and be reminded that they define IPE as 'occasions when two or more professions learn with, from and about each other to improve collaboration and the quality of care' (CAIPE 1997). This definition has been widely accepted and represents the standard to be achieved.

We are not convinced, however, that IPE per se will necessarily lead to collaborative working, especially if we are unclear as to its meaning.

So what exactly does collaboration really mean? According to the Oxford dictionary, it means 'teamwork, relationship, alliance' but is this all that IPE is hoping to achieve? Roschelle and Teasley (1995) suggest that collaboration '*is the motivational engagement of participants in a coordinated effort to solve a problem*'. For us the key word here is 'motivational'. If we use this definition, working collaboratively has to fundamentally involve cooperation among groups of professions, working within their own professional boundaries and expertise to solve a problem. It also means that we need to ensure that students and staff alike are motivated to work together – to see the benefits to themselves, their work and most importantly to their patient.

Whilst the CAIPE definition appears straightforward, how can we ensure that students learn to collaborate using Roschelle and Teasley's definition? There are many barriers to providing opportunities for students to learn with, from and about each other, both in practice and academia. The ultimate goal of IPE is to ensure that tomorrow's health and social care professionals have the skills, abilities and *motivation* to work together to deliver efficient, effective and quality patient-centred care, despite the challenges imposed by service needs and changes.

To achieve this, we have developed a model (Figure 10.1) built on our experiences of implementing IPE, which overcomes the many, and various, challenges associated with this type of learning. Our aim was to develop IPE which would increase students' and professionals'

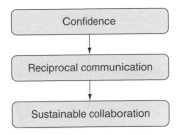

Figure 10.1   Key outcomes of IPE activity

confidence and belief in their own role, whilst also building their confidence and belief in others, thereby developing a trust, respect and value for their colleagues input in patient care. From our own experiences, we found that once students and staff had this confidence, the ability to communicate freely, honestly and without fear naturally occurred. This in turn broke down many barriers and preconceived stereotypes, resulting in positive and enjoyable work experiences, which benefited both patient and professional alike. We found that by working within this richer and more fulfilling interprofessional environment, those involved (especially students) gained a set of transferable skills which they took with them on to future placements.

Overcoming Challenges and the Birth of the Model

Whilst there are many models of IPE available (Lindqvist *et al.* 2005; O'Halloran *et al.* 2006; Lennox and Anderson 2007), the development, observation and evaluation of two models implemented by the authors form the basis for the Collaborative Model. We believe that this model highlights the infrastructure necessary for nurturing successful collaboration. Each step identifies factors needed to overcome implementation challenges found in practice and academic settings. The first activity: a virtual online patient pathway interwoven through a three year curriculum; and the second: an interprofessional practice based week. Both activities are reported in greater detail in Chapters 5 and 6.

These two types of IPE activity are very different in terms of size, timing, length, resources and environment, but we learned that they posed the same fundamental challenges for implementation.

Facing the Different Challenges

From an interprofessional learning (IPL) perspective, it is essential that the uniqueness and expertise of each profession is emphasised, and that it instils a respect and understanding of the different roles and responsibilities of others, as well as a recognition of potential collaborative working.

The variety and diversity of roles and responsibilities within health and social care professional groups serves to highlight the range of skills and expertise required to care for any one patient, service user or client. It goes without saying that no one professional group has the skills and expertise to provide total care for any one person. By working together, each profession should be able to join up all their skills and expertise to the patients benefit. As Gilbert (2005) states, *'The whole is greater than the sum of its parts.'* Yet, this is often the very area where IPE becomes unstuck. Today's climate of reduced resources and a stretched workforce contributes to professional instability and concern for role boundaries.

Perhaps, even before respect and understanding of contrasting roles can be instilled, one of the biggest challenges facing both practice- and higher education institution (HEI)-based IPE may be the logistical problems associated with the numbers of students, the variety of placements, the demand on human resource and the inequity of placement funding across the professions. In setting up IPL the biggest mistake can be to ignore these logistical challenges.

Whilst evidence suggests that students mostly prefer IPE in practice (partly, we reason because they are working and learning in the role and environment of their choosing), it may be easier, although not without its challenges, to deliver IPE within the academic environment. We wonder though, whether in this environment it might be more difficult to provide a 'real' collaborative experience for the students, which may be essential, if students are to be 'motivated' to work collaboratively. There are, however, perhaps more important reasons for delivering IPE in practice if we are to realistically provide students with the opportunity to practise what they learn and to bridge the gaps between learning and practice.

Higher Education Institutes, government and professional bodies may support and provide the thrust for IPE, but this may be of little value if demands within service are such that working uniprofessionally feels safer and more protected. During periods of stress and change it is likely that working uni- rather than interprofessionally will be favoured. Since the late 1980s workers in the National Health Service (NHS) have (and some would say, still are) experienced major change. We may, therefore, be in danger of providing students with the knowledge and skills to develop IPE but doom them to failure when we subject them to an environment where demands prevent them from working in this way. This may be one valid reason why IPE needs to be visible within workplaces and must involve frontline staff.

The use of a blended approach of virtual and practice IPE learning could ensure that students have an understanding of the roles, responsibilities and skills of their own and other professions prior to clinical practice, enabling them to put into practice this aspect of their learning easily and quickly, thereby allowing them to concentrate on learning to work collaboratively and to develop better patient care when in practice.

Creating the Model

Prior to implementation of any programme/activity, it is often necessary to consider and deal with covert issues, for example professional perspectives of the value of IPE to their own students, matters of time commitment and relevance to curricula. We found that the most successful way of dealing with these issues was to involve representatives from all professions, from the very beginning.

It is essential that visible support and leadership come from the heads of departments and clinical services involved in the IPE activity. It is at this level that the diverting of resources, disseminating of information to middle managers and credibility with other heads of departments, helps the initial challenge of introducing change. Once this is in place, it becomes possible to recruit champions (Figure 10.2), who will believe in the potential of IPE, have credibility within their own profession and be able to convince sceptical colleagues. They will also support each other which is especially important when faced with the surfeit of challenges surrounding IPE. Only two or three champions are needed per site to begin to explore the possibilities of what could be achieved through IPE. Working together champions are able to break down barriers, to develop ideas, to share the workload. One important point – we found most practitioners wanted to know that it had been cleared by their heads of the departments.

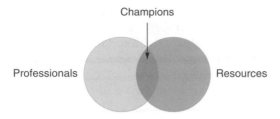

Creating the model

Figure 10.2   Step 1: Finding champions

An often overlooked area is that of resources. Inadequate resources make any task more difficult and can doom it to failure. We would, however, argue that there are a few essential resources, which are key to success. Dedicated and appropriate administrative support is essential to manage the many strands that invariably accompany IPE. The need to arrange meetings which suit all professionals involved in an IPE activity is vital; it is easy to fall at the first hurdle if individuals do not engage in the initial encounters. It is essential to pursue professionals to ensure engagement, and to demonstrate that they are valuable members of the team. Diaries need to be synchronised; the absence of clarity across the diaries of a range of individuals can have serious repercussions during an activity if one or more professional groups do not appear to be engaged. This can lead to reinforcement of stereotypes.

Appropriate rooms and resources need to be booked well ahead of time, to ensure planned IPE activities run smoothly in conducive settings. The smooth running of IPE activities require extra time, which most lecturers and practitioners do not have; their concerns and energies are channelled into uniprofessional concerns and interprofessional activities have a tendency, especially in the early phases of setting up to be seen as being an 'extra' piece of work, on top of their day-to-day responsibilities. It is essential, therefore, that dedicated support is available to develop and support the many layers of the activity. For online activities, a dedicated learning technologist is indispensable; their skills in responding quickly to any technical online issue is crucial; their ability to use the web space to create visual interactive pages that are engaging and inviting to both students and facilitators is essential. It is easy to underestimate the time and energy required to maintain engagement in an e learning environment; this, coupled with an interprofessional student audience, only serves to highlight the need for good technical support, as well as provision of training to develop good interprofessional e-facilitation skills.

Contacting and meeting with so many professionals can be time consuming, resource intensive and initially feel unsustainable. In hindsight, however, it reaps benefits.

Every profession is able to debate the advantages of the programme for their own students. It affords each professional group the opportunity to help shape and take part ownership of the programme. Following discussions with each professional group, natural champions begin to emerge and take the lead. Working together they are able to suggest activities which could work within the practice environment. They naturally choose activities where they know there will be sufficient resources available. This is a crucial factor, if long-term sustainability is to be achieved. Champions are an essential building block for this model.

Where champions do not emerge the challenges became insurmountable and the IPE activity, even if it manages to take place in the first instance, is not sustainable in the long term.

In such cases, we noted that when the week long activity commenced it became immediately apparent that there were pre-existing covert issues surrounding collaboration and teamworking among the permanent health and social care professionals on the ward.

Looking back at the number of difficulties experienced in this area, it is apparent that the length of time required preparing ward-based staff, prior to the introduction of students in an IPE activity, will vary dependent on a team's cohesiveness and integration. The better the team, the easier it is.

Variations between learners in terms of ability, age, prior educational achievement as well as clinical experience are frequently highlighted as barriers to IPE. Whilst recognising that each profession might cover identical topics uniprofessionally, the professional requirement of knowledge level in each subject varies immensely. However, IPE concerns the process of learning to work together, of learning to work collaboratively and as such relies more on a respect for the uniqueness of each profession, an understanding of where there is overlap and a recognition of how these similarities and differences can be used to the advantage of the patient and professional.

In our work we found that age, experience and prior education did not matter although this was not true in activities undertaken by Anderson and Thorpe (2008). We found that there were always gaps in each student's understanding of the other's profession irrespective of age or experience. What was crucial, however, was that students needed to feel safe and secure, free from any fear of ridicule and reassurance that no other team member would expect them to know everything. By ensuring that students were working in this environment we found that they were confident to ask questions which were key to increasing student confidence and resulted in growing respect and support across the team. It helped, of course, to pay attention to ground rules and to provide clear expectations for the group process, behaviour and access to help and support. Structured reflection which allowed everyone to contribute was also important (Headrick *et al.* 1998).

For pre-registration students (where most of our work occurred), there were major challenges associated with many academic policies – for example, type of assessment – whether it be a fail/pass, or modular or academic credit. Different universities have different policies and procedures as well as different rules of accreditation, different professional bodies and different guidelines; the logistics of working with more than one professional group, in addition to more than one university, certainly leads to periods of frustration, which may explain why IPE projects in the early days were often not sustained past an initial offering.

There are also major scheduling challenges, with professional groups having different semester/term lengths, beginning and end dates, different holidays, different scheduled placement and campus blocks, different exam schedules and exam boards, and a great variety of placement locations – some many miles away. The development of an online environment which enables students to work together in a virtual setting addresses the absence of physical proximity yet is often hampered by placement areas who fail to understand the importance of online learning and refuse students access to information systems. This obviously causes problems when students in practice are forced to complete IPE work in their own time. Whilst the students felt strongly about this, it was not the case for all lecturers, many of whom saw no difference in students undertaking work in their own time from any other module reading they might be expected to do. Other lecturers felt strongly that activities that had to be undertaken within a given period, and which were linked to assessment, should be given specific protected time, in the same way as one would be given time to attend a lecture or seminar. If students were in practice then time should be allocated within practice.

If learning to work in collaborative teams cannot be achieved through a single activity then there is a real need to agree when students should begin to participate in IPE. The debate as to whether IPE is better placed as a series of undergraduate or postgraduate activity continues. Advocates for postgraduate IPE activity consider that it is necessary to feel secure within one's own professional identity before being able to fully understand and work with other professionals. Others would advocate early exposure to IPE on the basis that professional stereotypes can diminish collaborative working. Recent evidence (Lindqvist *et al.* 2005) has shown that students start their professional courses with stereotypes of other professionals and that these stereotypes are often reinforced during their uniprofessional training. By introducing IPE early into professional training, it also supports the notion that IPE is not a one-off activity, but a part of lifelong learning (McPherson *et al.* 2001).

However, even when IPE is introduced early in the undergraduate curriculum as long as uniprofessional hierarchical structures exist, where IPE is viewed as a distraction and time taken from more important uniprofessional learning, difficulties will arise. It is crucial that these barriers are identified and addressed prior to implementing IPE programmes for there is little doubt that students are often influenced by the perspectives and beliefs of their teachers and mentors. Financial rewards and professional goals and competitiveness cannot be recognised in IPE in the same way as in uniprofessional education, making it an unwelcome and valueless activity for some.

Historical rivalries and fears of dilution of professional identities, not just across professions but within as well (e.g. branches of nursing, specialisms in medicine, between scientific and social-based professions), all serve to act as barriers to IPE.

Many professionals still harbour beliefs that IPE is no more than a covert method of deskilling professional groups and a threat to professional autonomy. Such perceptions can be very disabling and destructive. It is clear that the government policy initiatives discussed earlier in Chapters 1 and 2 have, in some cases, fostered a climate of mistrust. The Blair years of modernisation clearly led the development of extended roles, in particular for some nursing groups, which has led to unease in some areas, with professionals feeling that their roles are being whittled away. Understanding that IPE focuses on respecting and sharing of knowledge, of appreciating the skills and boundaries of each profession with its ultimate aim of working together to improve patient care is an important message to disseminate.

It is also imperative that students and professionals alike assume responsibility and are accountable for their actions; this requires an understanding of the limits and boundaries of their professional roles and autonomy to carry out their roles.

We have already identified that by meeting with professional groups a natural set of champions are born. McPherson *et al.* (2001) clearly highlight the commitment and time required to create and sustain IPE activities. This means that finding ways to create this time and to acknowledge the workload is essential if IPE is to be sustainable. Often IPE contributions are not recognised within university matrices or reward systems which focus on individual performance. Within practice, clinical staff who may have a reduced load by virtue of having a student still have to deal with the uncertainty of service needs within the NHS.

So why is it important in practice based (or in academia) learning that clinical practitioners create the IPE activity?

Students from different professions all undertake clinical practice in placement blocks, meaning that any one time there will be many students from different professions working in the same placement. It seems the most natural environment to develop IPE opportunities. It also provides students with the opportunity to participate as learners in a real life context where learning will make sense (Field 2004). Each student has a mentor and so naturally has an 'expert' in their own professional field. Learning outcomes specific to each student's placement will be available and need to be included within the IPL activity (clinical practitioners ensure that this occurs by developing the activity, Figure 10.3). In this way the activities within the IPE programme are

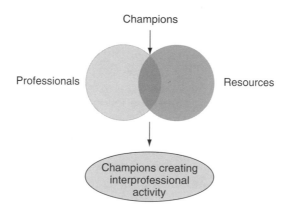

Figure 10.3 Creating the IPE activity

perceived as relevant to student and mentor/clinical practitioner both uniprofessionally and interprofessionally (McPherson *et al.* 2001).

The development of such applied and relevant IPE activities can be empowering if practitioners feel that they are addressing issues of patient care, using an activity they have created and therefore owned.

As mentioned earlier, champions tend to be a group of like-minded individuals able to support each other during times of frustration and difficulties. They have a basic knowledge and understanding, as well as a respect for the contributions of other members of the ward team.

This not only gives the activity credibility but also promotes ownership of the activity. We have found that this is the first step to ensuring the activity is sustainable (especially within practice, i.e. that it will continue without the need for long-term input from HEI). It makes sense that alongside the champions who carry the main load of both promoting IPE and engaging colleagues, there needs to be nominated leads for each IPE activity. Such leads need to be known, respected and trusted both within the IPE setting and within their uniprofessional context.

We found, however, that in the early days providing active support to these practitioners is crucial to success. Such support involves organising the meetings, working to their timetables, writing up the minutes, developing all the learning materials, providing templates which ensured that busy practitioners were able to simply pick up the paper-based information and 'run' with it. It is these extra 'administrative' aspects of establishing an activity which often prove to make the workload insurmountable. In practice the care of patients always takes priority. Recognising the competing demands on practitioners, in this way, can act as an enabler and empowerer. Practitioners are able to understand that this support will enable them to facilitate the activity without an inordinate amount of extra work and will help them find the energy to succeed.

Factors which cannot be predicted, but which we found impacted heavily on the implementation of IPE in practice, were the frequency of service setting changes occurring as a direct response to service demands – closure of wards, sudden change of duty rotas, movement of staff to cover other wards. We found that these sudden changes were more likely to occur within the larger acute hospitals and were hugely destructive not only for the IPE activity but for the students uniprofessional work, who were also subject to sudden changes – being moved into different specialties, moved onto nightshifts at short notice and given different mentors without discussion.

As referred to earlier in this chapter the stereotypical characteristics of specific groups have historically (and to some degree currently) been rife within the health and social care professions, not only across professions but also within professional specialisms. Negative as well as positive images can be found attached to any profession – for example, the notion that adult nurses have in the past been viewed as 'angels' by the general public or 'handmaids' by the doctors, or that surgeons possessed skills superior to those of general practitioners. Stereotypes such as these can very clearly impact on collaborative working. Negative stereotypes often come to the fore at times of conflict and can result in breakdown in communication. Within health and social care, there have been many cases of stereotyping through the misunderstanding of roles and responsibilities leading to catastrophes in individual's care, the case of Victoria Climbié being a clear example (Laming Report 2003).

Breaking down negative stereotypes is essential if IPE is to be successful. On a one-to-one level getting to know people as individuals may begin to break down negative beliefs/images held by both persons (it can, of course, cause the opposite and serve to reinforce especially if this meeting occurs at a time of conflict). Importantly, if IPE is placed within the context of working for a common goal, then it is more likely that working together as a team to achieve this goal will result in the breaking down of negative stereotypes and subsequently the affirmation of positive images (Burgess 2003). Using the patient/service user as the focus of any IPE (Figure 10.4) helps to overcome any preconceived ideas regarding different professionals – especially for students whose main aim is to care for and improve the outcome for every patient in their care.

Another important facet of using a patient is that all the clinical practitioners will have an input and role in the delivery of care. The patient acts as a focal point for each professional allowing for areas of learning to naturally occur for each student – for example, we found that use of language by different professions, often viewed as a mechanism for maintaining elitism, provided an area where each student could 'teach' the other students. Students were keen to be able to share their language with other students, demonstrating their understanding of their own body of knowledge. Something as simple as this proved to be a useful ice-breaker and a valuable aspect of learning between student groups.

Where students work in groups with a common goal (importantly patient-focused), supported by a group of committed practitioners or facilitators upon whom the students can call if they need, student communication and confidence both as an individual and as a team, both

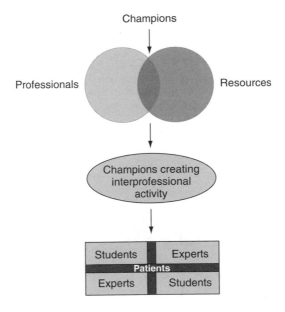

Figure 10.4 Using patients as the focal point of the learning activity

in their own professional role and in understanding the roles of others is clearly evident. (Figure 10.5)

We have also seen that the commitment and the enthusiasm of the student teams has an impact on the mentors (referred to as experts in the model – see Chapter 5), and facilitators who see the change not only in their own students but also students from other professions. As a result of the activity, mentors find that they communicate more than usual with other mentors who have students participating in the IPE activity. This increase in communication frequency, usually about the training needs of their students, brings them closer together. As the mentors gain confidence, they begin to work cooperatively to develop IPE activities which benefit all students, and which evaluation has shown (Chapter 5) benefits the patient.

At the beginning of the activity most students will work cooperatively as a team but as they communicate more and as their own confidence increases, they appreciate the need to work together cooperatively to deliver appropriate care to patients (Figure 10.6).

Students remark on the interdependence of their roles – where they overlap, how they can build on this for patient benefit and what changes

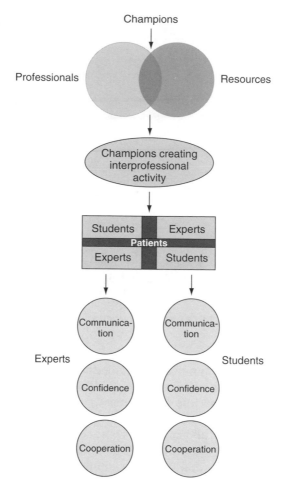

Figure 10.5 Communication and confidence grows: Learning process 2

they could suggest as 'newcomers' to the NHS. We believe that this learning is essential to facilitating attitude change in both students and mentors.

Student and professional evaluation of the activity is crucial to further development of the activity, to feed back to all participants and to all professional colleagues. In our experiences student and facilitator feedback contains many positive elements, feeding back these elements are

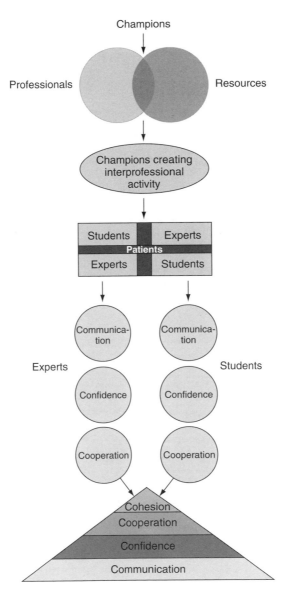

Figure 10.6 Cooperative working leads to cohesion within the team

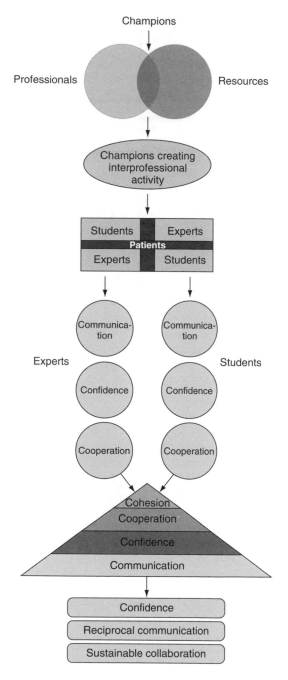

Figure 10.7 The collaborative model

key in creating a feeling of value, of positive outcome and of personal satisfaction – all important for developing ownership and sustainability.

IPE activities which last longer than 2 days allow students time to develop confidence and to begin to work cooperatively; feedback suggests that working in this way leads to increased satisfaction among staff and students and changes in daily routines. For example, students who normally worked 9–5 would come in at the beginning of shifts to participate in/observe the hand over between other professionals. Students began to look out for each other and to share lunch and coffee breaks.

The student's common focus of wanting to deliver quality care which meets the needs of their patients is evident and we believe is key to learning to understand and respect each other's roles. We believe that learning in this way naturally breaks down interprofessional barriers. We would suggest that through patient-focused care, be this face to face or via a virtual patient journey, students do begin to see the benefit, not only to the patient, but also to their own professional development of working interprofessionally. We believe that this encourages students to learn to become a more cohesive team player, who will be motivated to seek other students out to share and seek information, in a way they would not have done before.

In this model students and experts gain confidence and engage in reciprocal communication – both of which are key to sustainability and which result in collaborative working. Collaborative working is an essential aspect of interprofessional working. We believe that students who have participated in the IPE activities we offer not only learn how to work cooperatively, but more importantly are willing to collaborate. Our evidence is based on seeing students actively seeking each other out to share information not only during the activity but in their feedback of how it has changed their practice. In this way students could be in the forefront of collaborative working through collaborative learning (Figure 10.7).

Conclusion

This chapter highlights a few of the challenges we and others have experienced when implementing IPE. The challenges are similar for most people, irrespective of the location, length or type of IPE. We have put forward a model which we believe highlights fundamental elements necessary, if the ultimate aim of IPE is to improve work in collaboration and consequently the quality of care given to patients/users. IPE activities need to act as a driving force to instil in health and social care professionals the belief that working together as a team is the only way to achieve patient/user-focused care which results in improved quality of care for that patient/user.

IPE programmes/activities can provide students with the understanding of each other's roles and responsibilities, a respect for each other's professional roles and responsibilities and an understanding of the uniqueness and overlap of each professional's roles – but will this result in the motivation to engage with others? We would suggest that the key word for all IPE is 'motivational engagement' and if we replace 'solve a problem' with 'achieve patient and family centred goals' then IPE is aiming to instil in all students the 'desire to engage with others' and to view this as an integral aspect of their professional behaviour. Perhaps this is where the real challenge lies and why we should continue to address the challenges and barriers which seem to be common to many IPE activities within planning, implementing and sustaining.

For us, this practice based IPE week is now a functioning aspect of one placement and runs as a result of the permanent team of ward-based health and social care professions. It is sustainable and offers a small group of students the opportunity to work as an IPE student team safely but to some degree independently.

References

Anderson, E. and L. Thorpe. (2008). Early interprofessional interactions: Does student age matter? *Journal of Interprofessional Care* 22 (3), 263–282.

Barker, K.K., C. Bosco and I.F. Oandasan. (2005). Factors in implementing interprofessional education and collaborative practice initiatives: Findings from key informant interviews. *Journal of Interprofessional Care* 19 (S1), May, 166–176.

Burgess, Heidi. (2003). 'Stereotypes/Characterization Frames', in *Beyond Intractability*, Guy Burgess and Heidi Burgess (eds). Boulder: Conflict Research Consortium, University of Colorado. Posted: October 2003, http://www.beyondintractability.org/essay/stereotypes/. Accessed 22 February 2008.

CAIPE. (1997) 'Interprofessional Education – A Definition', *CAIPE Bulletin* 13, 19.

Field, D. (2004). Moving from novice to expert – the value of learning in clinical practice: A literature review. *Nurse Education* 24, 560–565.

Gilbert, J.H.V. (2005). Interprofessional learning and higher education structural barriers. *Journal of Interprofessional Care* 19 (S1), 87–106.

O'Halloran, C., S. Hean, D. Humphris and J. Macleod-Clark. (2006). Developing common learning: The new generation project undergraduate curriculum model. *Journal of Interprofessional Care* 20 (1), 12–28.

Headrick, L.A., P.M. Wilcock and P.B. Batalden. (1998). Interprofessional working and continuing medical education. *BMJ* 316 (7133), 771–774.

Jackson, J.A. and P.A.S. Bluteau. (2007). At first it's like shifting sands: Setting up interprofessional learning within a secondary care setting. *Journal of Interprofessional Care* 21 (3), June, 351–353.

Laming Report. (2003). *The Victoria Climbié Inquiry.* Presented to the Secretary of State for Health and the Secretary for the Home Department.

Lennox, A. and E.S. Anderson. (2007). *The Leicester Model of Interprofessional Education: A Practical Guide to Implementation in Health and Social Care Education.* Special Report 9. The Higher Education Academy Subject Centre for Medicine, Dentistry and Veterinary Medicine.

Lindqvist, S., A. Duncan, L. Shepstone, F. Watts and S. Pearce. (2005). Case-based learning in cross-professional groups – the development of a pre-registration interprofessional learning programme. *Journal of Interprofessional Care* 19 (5), 509–520.

McPherson, K., L. Headrick and F. Moss. (2001). Working and learning together: Good quality care depends on it, but how can we achieve it? *Quality in Health Care* 10 (Suppl. 2), ii, 46–53.

Roschelle, J. and S. Teasley. (1995). 'The construction of shared knowledge in collaborative problem solving', in *Computer Supported Collaborative Learning,* C.E. O'Malley (ed.). Heidelberg: Springer-Verlag, pp. 69–97.

11

Sustaining Interprofessional Education in Professional Award Programmes

Marilyn Hammick and Elizabeth Anderson

Introduction

In this chapter we discuss the sustainability of interprofessional education (IPE).[1] By this we mean an enduring acceptance that continuous cohorts of students will learn about interprofessionalism and will learn interprofessionally within their professional[2] education programme. Our purpose is to spotlight reasons why embedding interprofessional learning in curricula is important and challenging.

The arguments we develop have a dual focus. First, the long-term integration of interprofessionalism with the other topics in the curriculum. This means ensuring its place, and achieving visible links between interprofessionalism, the social sciences and professional practice on the curriculum map. Second, the acceptance of interprofessional learning as a means towards competence and capability in interprofessional practice and collaborative working. Our interest is in what may enable, and can disable, the sustainability of change and innovation in professional education, especially where these processes introduce learning styles and topics that are contested.

We have taken our lead in planning what to write, by reflecting first on the title of the opening chapter of this book. This choice was based on our conviction that successful pilots encourage further interprofessional learning initiatives. From there, we discuss what professional education (in particular for this book in health and social care but not exclusively) might look like if IPE was a normative part of all UK undergraduate programmes that lead to registration with an appropriate UK statutory registration body. Our hope is that our international readership can translate this parochial wish for their local situation.

The questions that underpinned our reflections were as follows:

- What does it mean for a given topic to be embedded in an educational programme?
- What will be the nature and content of curricula that have interprofessionalism and collaborative practice as embedded topics?
- What impact will sustained IPE have on students and staff?
- What issues arise during the process of developing and mainstreaming IPE in any professional education or training programme?

After the Beginning

As Chapter 1 suggests many interprofessional learning initiatives begin in a small way. Increasingly, this type of beginning is officially recognised as pilot work, signalling an intention to assess the impact of the initial work and to use findings from that, to develop and integrate the new programme or course with existing curricula. To establish some context for this final chapter, we drew upon our personal knowledge of IPE that began in this very way: as pilots that were evaluated, modified and have subsequently been part of the curriculum for ongoing cohorts of students.

Boxes 11.1–11.3 highlight the key features of these examples of maintained IPE. We have rather deliberately identified differences in both the curriculum models and key features related to the development in a particular location. Taking the local context into account and developing *your* model of IPE is a key mechanism of effectiveness (Hammick *et al.* 2007). This is an important message for staff responsible for developing and sustaining IPE. It is possible to learn from and in part to replicate good models: they (almost) always need to be adapted to the local context. So, please read this chapter from the perspective of your local situation. We are not advocating conformity. Knowing what to disregard from the following discussion is as important as identifying what is key in your particular educational setting.

The examples in Boxes 11.1–11.3 could provoke an argument that this chapter is redundant; that we are pessimists by acknowledging the need to discuss sustainability. Our first response to that is to applaud the staff and institutions where IPE has been maintained and where

Box 11.1 A UK Community based Model of IPE

The practice based Health in the Community model was designed with and for medical students to study the complexities of delivering patient-centred care in a multidisciplinary setting where health inequalities were greatest. Its original community setting reflected the need to address the imbalance in medical education between hospital and community care (Lennox and Petersen 1998). The model engages higher education institutions in partnership with all aspects of service. The stages of the model and cycle of learning enable experiential, problem-based reflective learning. Led by patients, it propels students, teachers and practitioners into a cycle of analysis leading towards a richer appreciation of the realities of teamworking and collaboration. This model has been sustained over ten years following long-term research evidence demonstrating value (Lennox and Anderson 2007). The first interprofessional learning pilot events began in 1998 with 24 medical students and 12 nursing students. By 2005, there were 14 clinical psychology students, 185 undergraduate and 65 graduate medical students, 83 nurses, 23 pharmacy students, 89 social work students and 50 speech and language therapy students. Today this course is integrated into the curriculum and involves 700+ students a year as part of the Leicestershire, Northamptonshire and Rutland (now the South Trent Health Authority) Interprofessional Education Strategy (Anderson and Knight 2003).

Box 11.2 Further Development of IPE Opportunities

Opportunities to increase the practice areas where the model described in Box 11.1 could be delivered led, in 1998, to learning focussed on the experiences of disabled people and a module entitled 'Learning from Lives' (Anderson *et al.* 2003). This enabled medical students to experience the work of rehabilitation teams in community hospitals where disability and equality issues are paramount. Particularly important in this initiative was the involvement of an organisation of people with disabilities, Leicestershire Centre for Integrated Living (LCIL), which enabled students to be brought face to face with the perspectives of disabled people. Following successful delivery of this module over a number of years, a successful funding bid provided an extension to include social work students in 2006: this made the experience truly interprofessional (Smith and Anderson 2006). Positive evaluation of these early initiatives has led to a wider range of students, from the allied health professions and nursing, into programmes where in interprofessional teams they learn to care for the disabled. These learning opportunities are now part of the local IPE aspects of professional curriculum.

Box 11.3 A UK-based Pilot IPE Initiative and Its Development

An evidence-based IPE initiative involving first year undergraduate students studying medicine, nursing, physiology and occupational therapy was initially piloted. Campbell's phased approach and complexity theory guided the development of the initiative and its evaluation. The work included a staff training programme, e learning materials and interprofessional teamworking skills workshops. A multi-method study design was used to evaluate the outcomes and the process of the initiative. A first year cohort of 442 students was invited to attend and 54% accepted. Findings showed that the intervention promoted theoretical learning about teamworking. It enabled the students to learn with and from each other; it significantly raised awareness about collaborative practice, and its links to improving the effectiveness of care delivery. Qualitative data results showed that the initiative increased students' confidence in their own professional identity and helped them to value difference, thus making them better prepared for clinical placement. This IPE is now compulsory and the project has evolved to include trained service users/carers as co-facilitators by integrating the generic material into the curricula of all professional courses. (Cooper *et al.* 2005)

---

evaluation continues as part of good educational practice. Second, we counter the redundancy argument with a note of caution about the curriculum hierarchy and with a discussion of *real* sustainability.

Interprofessionalism and the Curriculum[3] Hierarchy

Opportunities for interprofessional learning have been available for a relatively short time in the long history of professional education programmes. Compare, for example, the longevity of bio-mechanics in physiotherapy, anatomy in medical education, radiation sciences in diagnostic and therapeutic radiography, and sociology and psychology in social work programmes. Of course, the age of a topic should not and does not give it a predestined right to be in the curriculum. However, standing the test of time, being there after the regular and searching curriculum reviews, now undertaken by the numerous statutory and regulatory bodies every five, or in some cases three, years, confers an element of worthiness on a topic. In addition, where subject benchmarking is used to denote good practice, the inclusion of that topic in these quasi-official documents gives it a gravitas that can make it harder to remove it, or even to just reduce its weight in the curriculum.

Reviews of education programmes often encounter the cyclical process of including the latest, very good and necessary topic as a subset of the curriculum, until another topic with equal importance, but with perhaps, more contemporary reasons for being there comes along. A change of government, yet another crisis in the delivery of care and well-being services, and a bright young thing from a radical think tank may have another solution to criticisms of the frequently beleaguered public services. Learning together, to work better together, may be pushed aside by this latest response.

New topics are also at risk from the regular call for the return to learning more of the basics, for example the natural sciences in medicine. Such calls are not simply asking for a return to the past but also advocate new teaching and learning methods, for example body painting for anatomy (McMenamin 2007). This makes one more call on time, which is precious in any curriculum.

We cannot imagine a topic of greater value to professional practice as that of learning to work collaboratively with other members of the service delivery team. It makes absolute sense to us that students should learn how to deliver their particular aspects of care and well-being with their peers from other professions, who are also members of the service team. We are convinced that learning about those *others* and from them leads to *learning with each other*, enabling a deeper understanding from all professional perspectives about the delivery of care services. This conviction is increasingly shared by many others but sceptics remain and many question the effectiveness of interprofessional learning.

The delivery of more effective care and well-being services to individuals and the community is unarguably the ultimate desired outcome of interprofessional learning. Of equal importance as measures of effectiveness are changes in knowledge, attitudes and skills, and subsequent changes in practice-related behaviours. There is evidence to support the effectiveness of IPE when measured against this range of outcomes (Barr *et al.* 2005; Hammick *et al.* 2007). Evidence about the mechanisms that lead to the provision of effective IPE also exists (Hammick *et al.* 2007). However, the absolute weight of this evidence is light. It is a truism that there are more calls for evidence that interprofessional learning *works* than for many other recently introduced curriculum changes in professional education!

The changes outlined above not only mean new curriculum content that includes interprofessionalism but also mean a change in the learning process to enable authentic interprofessional learning. In other words, the curriculum needs to include new topics (about interprofessionalism, for example, what constitutes effective teamworking) *and* interactive ways of delivering this learning. It is unsurprising in these circumstances that achieving the rightful place of interprofessionalism in a particular curriculum is a challenge.

We turn now to the matter of identifying what an interprofessional curriculum and interprofessional learning might look like. After all, a *visible* goal is more likely to be achieved.

Mapping the Interprofessional Curriculum

The topics (anatomy, etc.) in particular curricula previously given as examples are truly integrated into the curriculum because they provide a necessary foundation for subsequent topics. These subsequent topics are enduring and essential elements of professional knowledge. A map of the curriculum would show a logical and indisputable route from the basic science to the applied science and to professional practice.

In radiography, knowledge of how radiation interacts with matter enables radiography students to learn the skill of selecting the optimum settings for a fit for purpose radiograph. That radiograph, in turn, leads to a diagnostic decision that contributes to patient care. In medicine, students study biomedical sciences – (physiology, anatomy with biochemistry, genetics, pharmacology, biophysics, biomedical engineering, molecular biology, cell biology) to understand how the body works, in order to understand the relationship between pathology and clinically presenting signs and symptoms. A historical glimpse at radiography and medical undergraduate curriculum maps would show the points given above as ever present (Weatherall 2006). However, not all topics remain in situ permanently; quite rightly, what is in any curriculum is regularly contested.

For example, tracking changes in UK medical education, we can see that in 1993 the General Medical Council (GMC) said, '*the burden of factual information imposed on students in undergraduate medical curricula should be substantially reduced*' (GMC 1993:23). Ten years later their report, Tomorrows Doctors, further reduced the requirement for basic science education (GMC 2003). These decisions may at any time be reversed, especially if there is evidence of doctor's problem-solving abilities being compromised.

Cyclical changes such as these can also be traced in nurse education where the basic science content has also fluctuated over the years. Our point here is that the pressures in a curriculum are multiple. They create competition between old and new topics, of which one is learning to be interprofessional. Attempts to introduce novel topics and new ways of learning need to be done with the cognisance of what curriculum change involves.

One response to the need for new topics is, understandably, that in current overcrowded curricula if one topic is to be added, then something has to be removed. This is not something we believe always has to happen in respect of IPE but it is helpful to hold that thought for a moment. Try to imagine the reaction to the suggestion that some of the basic sciences should be removed from the curriculum they are part of, and you can understand how well rooted these are in healthcare sciences curricula. We are not suggesting by this that these topics are removed: we are simply demonstrating what being embedded means.

That said, as with the garden rose, regular and expert pruning of curriculum is wise. It leads to renewed vigour and a curriculum that stays well. It provides the opportunity for new topics, of which interprofessional matters are important ones, the opportunity to take root and grow. Careful thought by all stakeholders, leading to judicious changes, guards against stagnation and complacency as Freeth (2001) reminds us. We also need to take the same critical stance with the interprofessional topics, whether recent or well established in a curriculum.

It follows from our comment about the basic science examples given above that for IPE to become embedded in a curriculum we need to map the logical route from learning the fundamentals of interprofessionalism to the end point of contributing to patient or client care. This is different from and complementary to establishing evidence for the effectiveness of interprofessional learning. Its focus is on logic and knowledge processes rather than simplistically on outcomes. Presently, the links between fundamental and well-understood sociological *and* psychological processes *and* learning interprofessionally and professional practice behaviour is somewhat atheoretical. Scholarly work to build concepts and models of interprofessional learning from empirical work is essential to its survival.

We now turn to more recent additions to professional curricula that are now (almost) as well embedded as topics from the natural sciences. For example, that part of the curriculum that covers professional values and competencies. We believe there is a case to be made for elaboration of and additionality to the professionalism curriculum: leading naturally to the development of a separate and equally essential interprofessional curriculum. But why a separate curriculum and why is it essential?

We would argue that for practitioners who are going to deliver effective public services in the twenty-first century, learning how *to be* interprofessional is as necessary as learning how *to be* a professional (McNair 2005; Wynd 2003). The values and beliefs of each profession are shaped by its unique customs and practices: learning what it means to be a nurse is fundamental to being a nurse and is different to learning what it means to be a social worker (Bernd *et al.* 2005; Brockopp *et al.* 2003). Readers of this book will be familiar with these differences and aware of the overlap between the professional attributes of these practitioners and the many other examples we could give. That place of overlap and the reality of public service delivery as a collaborative endeavour have given rise to interprofessional customs and practices and a set of unique interprofessional values and beliefs. Conflating professionalism and interprofessionalism can only serve to confuse; each deserves its rightful place as a topic in professional programmes (Evetts 1999).

Our argument is for a postmodern perspective on those attributes that contribute to services and practice being delivered in the right way. In other words, a celebration of difference and recognition that professionalism cannot be generalised to the new and different ways of twenty-first-century working. We would go further to assert that practitioners who know what to do, and yet not know how to do that interprofessionally, are not fit for purpose in the twenty-first-century health and social care milieu. The shift towards partnership models of health and social care delivery, and between service users and their health and social care providers, reinforces the need for additional and interprofessional attributes.

Preparation of future practitioners needs to focus on ways that guard against the tendency of uniprofessionalism to create insularity and to support the sense of the power and control of one profession. In its place there is a collective responsibility to encourage interprofessionalism with its heightened sense of altruism and less self-interest. To date, aspects of interprofessionalism, for example, the ability to cooperate with others is frequently defined as a small part of effective professionalism and for many health and social care professions defining what constitutes professionalism is an on-going debate (Hilton and Slotnick 2005; Jha *et al.* 2007). But a sustainable interprofessional curriculum cannot be part of something else; it needs to be a separate entity and it is this that we focus on next by asking

What are the features of the interprofessional curriculum map, where learning to work together in routine and novel situations has equal rights in the timetable, as the examples given above?

Put another way, what would IPE look like if staff no longer had to make *special* arrangements for students to have opportunities for inter-professional learning? In this situation the curriculum would naturally include these, as much as it did opportunities to experience learning about all the other basic and essential professional attributes. We want to show what topics might be included in the interprofessional syllabus that would make it complementary to the professionalism syllabus. Two processes (at least) are involved in this change: reforming topics presently included and adding new topics.

Reformation

Our first example, here, relates to knowledge and skilful use of com-munication. It is no longer necessary for students to simply develop an understanding of the role of communication with and about patients, clients and family caregivers within the scope of their professional practice and the necessary attitudes and skills to foster effective com-munication between their peers (intraprofessional communication). It is also essential for them to understand and be competent at interprofes-sional communication. This example is one where it could be said that an extension to what is already in the curriculum is needed. In this way, the topic of communication is elaborated to be fit for purpose for tomorrow's practitioners.

Evidence to support the need for this elaboration can be found in the report of the enquiry into the care of Victoria Climbié. This cites poor quality interprofessional communication throughout the care of this young child (Laming Report 2003). In his report Lord Laming espe-cially stressed the need for processes and mechanisms for the exchange of information between those from different professions. Writing at that time Revans (2002) reported that '*as phase one of the Victoria Climbié Inquiry ended this week, a picture was emerging of professions that simply do not understand each other*'. Learning about each other addresses this deficit.

One recommendation of the Laming Report (see Box 11.4) provides an insight into one of the key issues of interprofessional communication: that of sharing, with practitioners from other professions, information about a service user. It is not only about what to share, but also about

---

**Box 11.4 From the Laming Report, Part Six:
Recommendations, p. 373**

'The Government should issue guidance on Data Protection Act 1998, and
the Human Rights Act 1998, and common rules on confidentiality. The government should issue guidance as when these impact on the sharing of
information between professional groups in circumstances where there are
concerns about the welfare of children and families'.

---

when to exchange confidential material between professional groups.
The constant tendency for separate professional record keeping continues to exacerbate this problem. As the Laming Report highlighted, the
historical barriers to the exchange of information are in need of attention at governmental level. However, even with legislation this remains
problematic, and the introduction of the dilemmas it raises merits a
place in initial health and social care education programmes.

Other examples of behaviours included in the professionalism syllabus include respect for others and team membership skills. Both these
can look and feel very different in an intraprofessional setting compared to that where practitioners from other professions participate. The
inability to see past historical hierarchies and stereotypical views of practitioners from the 'other' professions can engender arrogance or a lack
of confidence: learning about each other provides the opportunity for
myths to be dispelled. Similarly, we cannot assume that team membership skills transfer easily from, for example, the traditional medical firm
or physiotherapy ward team to the rehabilitation team responsible for a
patient with long-term care needs. Today and tomorrow's public service
workers need to learn the basic skills of how to work in the interprofessional team within the relatively comfortable setting of their initial
education programme.

Addition

We continue with a discussion of the need for additional topics in the
curriculum, so that students have the opportunity to learn how to be
interprofessional. Box 11.5 has examples of how the delivery of services
is shaped by interprofessional collaborative practice.

These new ways of working mean that practitioners need to respect
difference and celebrate this in daily practice. This interprofessional
attribute that can so clearly benefit service users is key to achieving

Box 11.5 Examples of Collaborative Practice

- Piertroni establishing a unique multidisciplinary healthcare centre in Marylebone, London, blending alternative therapies within health and social care (Pietroni, R. and Pietroni, C. 1995).
- Dr Angela Lennox working to bring together services to overcome poverty and deprivation in Leicester (NHS Beacon practices 2000).
- Pen Green Centre in Corby Northamptonshire, which opened in 1993 for under 5s and their families, led by a multidisciplinary team and jointly managed by Education, Social Services and the local Health Authority (Whalley, M., 2001; www.pengreen.org.uk).

high-quality collaborative care. It is no longer just necessary for practitioners to be capable and competent within their domains of professional practice. In addition to excellent one-to-one care between practitioner and service user, all staff need to work interprofessionally. There is widespread acceptance that learning about others, from others and with others provides a sound base for effective collaborative working. This way of learning is, of course, valuable at any time in a practitioner's working life. IPE continues as part of service improvement initiatives leading to changes that make a real difference to patient and client care. However, the focus in this book is on initial professional education programmes: it is to the additions to the curriculum for learners on these programmes that we now turn.

By heading this section *addition* we are not necessarily advocating that this means putting a great deal extra in the curriculum. Enabling interprofessional learning is as much about how it is done as it is about the subjects that are learnt. We believe it is important that interprofessional learning in initial education programmes is logical and gentle; logical because of the complexity of moving into a new genre of learning; gentle because of the delicate balance needed between learning to be a (particular) type of professional practitioner and learning to be interprofessional. In this way learning to understand and respect the 'otherness' of others becomes a valuable and interesting aspect of professional education, and not a threat to the future role of the student.

The logic is supplied by moving from learning about each other, from each other and then with each other within an authentic context. This may be in the workplace, in a clinical skills laboratory or with simulated patients. It can also be achieved through case-based, enquiry- or problem-based learning on the campus: and by a combination of workplace- and campus-based learning. In many places the numbers of students involved in IPE mean that imaginative and innovative blended learning is used. For example, some initial face-to-face group work continued as e learning as students follow the classroom/work-placement model in their uniprofessional course. In this way interprofessional learning takes its rightful place alongside uniprofessional learning: gently introducing students to the importance of knowing how to work collaboratively within the context of also learning to be a social worker, a physiotherapist a . . .

An interprofessional curriculum offers the opportunity to explore traditional and new roles within health and social care, especially related to wider concepts of health as well-being, rather than as ill-health. In this way, students become more aware of their limits of competence and of the competence of others. The aim is a firmer appreciation of where the expertise of one profession stops, that of another begins, and the opportunity to learn the first post competences needed for collaborative working. In this way, IPE provides the foundation for newly qualified staff to be able to effectively participate in what Meads and Ashcroft (2005:7) write as the 'three pillars of (inter) professional accountability', namely 'risk assessment, performance management and (evidence-based) quality improvement'.

Importantly, these authors focus on the positive drivers for learning and working together in making their case for interprofessional collaboration. This is particularly relevant at a time when services are being reconfigured, health and other statutory sector budgets pooled, and community well-being services redesigned as models of partnership working between diverse public sector service providers (DoH 2001; DfES 2004). Meads and Ashcroft (2005) also remind us of the role of learning to work together in crisis prevention. It is not our intention to do more than reference the strong arguments well made in that text. We recommend the case studies of the enquiries led by Laming and Kennedy as essential reading for anyone who remains unconvinced of the need for interprofessional learning and working within the context of safeguarding the public.

Both enquiries mentioned above remind us that the reality of the workplace and the complexities of service delivery are intricate, challenging and carry the potential for critical, even catastrophic failure. The educational response to this must be fit for purpose.

In this section we have argued that learning interprofessionally and interprofessional learning need a concrete and continuing place in initial education curricula, which aim to prepare students for work in most, if not all, public services. This includes health and social services and many of the other services that promote and support well-being. We don't believe these essential components can just as easily be learnt uniprofessionally. The future workforce requires preparation for their collaborative roles in learning situations that are authentic, and reflect the reality of the workplace. Students need opportunities like this to learn about the principles underpinning being interprofessional, and how these theoretical concepts relate to collaborative practice. In this way learning leads to understanding of the skills and attitudes needed to work interprofessionally; and thus to competence in collaborative working.

Finally, preparation for effective interprofessional practice depends upon a personal and professional responsibility to reflect on care or actions taken. Schön (1987) argued that competent practice relies on reflection-in-action – *the ability to monitor what one is doing as one is doing it* – and reflection-on-action – *the ability to reflect on one's actions and to translate this reflection back into the practice*. Students need to be enabled to self-examine, and are frequently given tools to help them develop these skills from within a professional domain (Moon 1999). However, the true mark of a highly competent interprofessional practitioner is the ability to reflect not just within a professional domain, but across professional domains. Only when professionals have the ability to reflect interprofessionally can they ever seek to become transformative in all aspects of practice. This type of ability is what hallmarked the leaders of the developments in Box 11.5. Developing this ability requires opportunities to learn from and about, and learn and work with, other practitioners (including those in the voluntary and community sectors) throughout a career span. Such learning enables reflection with those who see the world of health and social care differently, challenge the status quo and advance and improve care (Wackerhausen 2007).

Measuring the Achievement of Interprofessionalism

We now turn our attention to measuring student attainment of competence in being an interprofessional practitioner. Our contention is that the achievement of learning how to be interprofessional should be assessed in the same way as all other topics in an undergraduate or initial education curriculum. Space limits a full discussion of this important aspect. We simply highlight below some reasons why 'interprofessional' should be assessed and some of the challenges associated with assessment of interprofessional learning.

Reasons

Assessment of competence in any aspect of professional practice should be driven by the recognition that practitioners who have this capability will be fit for purpose. It follows that without such competence the service they deliver will be less than optimal. Interprofessional competence should be measured because we have a responsibility to ensure that first post practitioners have the knowledge and skills to work collaboratively, to reflect on service user outcomes, from within their own and other professional perspectives, and to apply their interprofessional skills in the right way. In other words, they know why they should be interprofessional and how to behave interprofessionally. This is recognised by many of the professional and regulatory bodies as the examples in Table 11.1 show. Each uses a different form of words and arguably has a different emphasis. However, the message is clear and is echoed by other bodies not cited here: students should learn how to work collaboratively and their ability to do so should be measured.

Table 11.1   Professional Body Guidance and Requirements Related to Learning to Be Collaborative: Three Examples

Professional body	Guidance and requirements
General Medical Council: Tomorrows Doctors 2003	Graduates must be aware of current developments and guiding principles in the NHS, for example,
	f) *the importance of working as a team within a multiprofessional environment*
Nursing and Midwifery Council (2007): Standards of proficiency for pre-registration nursing education to register	Demonstrate knowledge of effective interprofessional working practices with respect and utilise the contributions of members of the health and social care team
National Occupational Standards for Social Work (2002)	Key Role Three: requires social workers to develop and maintain professional relationships within and outside the organisation; to work within multidisciplinary teams and multi-organisational team, networks and systems (Unit 22); and to establish and maintain effective working relationships within and outside the organisation (Unit 23)

This raises the issue of students' perceptions of topics in any curriculum that are not assessed. We are not suggesting that non-assessment of a topic has a direct relationship with how the learner approaches it. After all, it is foolish to think that everything can be assessed. Our point is related to the strength of importance attached to any part of the syllabus that is clearly not going to be assessed (Race 2005). Whilst it remains challenging, measuring interprofessional competence must be faced, if learners are going to accept its importance in their crowded curriculum.

Challenges

We have argued about the responsibility of ensuring that first post practitioners have the knowledge and skills to work collaboratively, and that they apply their interprofessional skills in the right way. There is an increasing body of knowledge about what this knowledge should consist of, what skills are needed and what attitudes enable the optimal application of these skills. Individual programmes with some experience in teaching and assessing an interprofessional curriculum have an increasing body of knowledge to share on this. Outside these international beacon sites, less is known and little is agreed on what should be assessed and perhaps, even less about how to assess interprofessional competencies. The first challenge for all of us is a discussion, and some agreement about what should be assessed and how it should be assessed. We are not suggesting rules here, simply a framework that permits a sensible level of parity across different programmes. We are also cognisant of the lack of a real consensus concerning how to assess the related topic of professionalism (Deirdre *et al.* 2004).

One aspect, needing attention, is the challenge of assessing the individual *skill* of teamwork alongside assessment of *knowledge*. For example, knowledge of interprofessional referral pathways, the achievement of effective user-centred interprofessional management plans, theoretical appreciation of the constituents in team dynamics, such as an ability to lead. In addition, and perhaps even more difficult, is the need to assess *attitudes* or having a positive regard of the values of interprofessional practice.

Issues arise about whether or not these assessments should be done in interprofessional student group settings and if so who should do the assessment. One example of assessed teamworking comes from Swedish training wards where interprofessional teaching and assessment has been sustained over several decades. Here students in the final stages of training are assessed in action by competent senior clinicians and team members as part of their clinical practice (Fallsberg and Wijma 1999; Fallsberg and Hammar 2000).

If we are to move towards interprofessional student group assessment, there will be a need for the aligning of the cultural gaps between the academic traditions involved *and* new agreements within academia and by professional bodies. The policy imperatives on collaboration compel agreement about how to measure interprofessionalism and ensure meaningful weighting of the topic within summative assessment schemes. Agreement is also needed about external examiner review of interprofessional assessments and a system of appropriate expert review of the interprofessional curriculum by the professional, statutory and regulatory bodies.

A way forward

Portfolios, which enable students to collect evidence of knowledge and experience with direct observations of skills and attitudes by peers or supervisors, remain an important starting point for assessing interprofessional competence, despite issues of consistency and comparability. These types of assessment tools will be welcomed by employers struggling to differentiate between candidates. Students who can turn to collective assessed evidence on their interprofessional competence may soon be the successful candidate for the sought-after job. Indeed, employers may become strong drivers for the sustainability of IPE through their demand for assessed evidence. Already newly qualified doctors cannot begin to find employment without first completing a reflective account to demonstrate *'how they work in a team'* (DoH 2003). Much more is needed in this respect.

Impact of the Interprofessional Curriculum

Our introduction indicated the need to keep the interests of key stakeholders in the education process in mind during curriculum change process. The next section looks briefly at what embedding interprofessionalism in the curriculum means for students and workplace and campus teaching staff.

Students

Evidence continues to suggest that students arrive from secondary education with deeply ingrained and historically informed views, about what it is to be a particular health and social care practitioner (Hean *et al.* 2006). Evidence suggests that negative stereotypical views can be mediated through effective IPE (Cooper *et al.* 2005; Anderson and Thorpe 2008). Rather naturally, students are at first hesitant and unsure of interprofessional learning, but many become enthusiasts for this and for interprofessional working. Student voices helped to evolve the Leicester Model of Interprofessional Education by reflecting on those aspects which caused problems to some groups of students, for example medical phrases in workbooks.

Interprofessional student networks that enable students to shape the future of interprofessional learning thrive in Canada and the UK. More may be in operation by the time this book is published. When these students graduate, they will become change agents and effective ambassadors for sustaining IPE. Indeed, sustaining IPE may depend (in part) on robust studies that identify and disseminate the student voice. More should and could be done to include students in curriculum design and delivery processes. See, for example, the Leicester Model where students were asked to influence the evolving new learning experience (Box 11.6).

Thoughtful introductory sessions that enable students to understand the relationship between learning together and their future practice as a member of the collaborative service delivery team have been shown to help to ease learners into the very different world of interprofessional learning (Box 11.7). Postgraduate students on interprofessional courses benefit from a discussion about the theoretical basis of the challenges groups of learners from different professional and disciplinary backgrounds face. Knowing why learning with their colleagues feels uncomfortable at times, via an understanding of the uniqueness of particular ontologies and epistemologies, is something to be leant on when the learning with others gets tough.

Box 11.6 Student Involvement in Course Development

A proposed structure by the authors on problem based principles was presented to members of student and staff committees and to 16 1st and 2nd Year students. The purpose of the course and its place in the curriculum was explained. Students understood that they were to refine the course ... the students input helped us to refine the course. (From Lennox and Petersen 1998, pp. 596–598)

Box 11.7 Introducing Students to Interprofessional Learning

In launching a new interprofessional strategy in 2005, Universities in Leicester-shire, Northamptonshire and Rutland invested £10,000 in designing a short film to depict why the interprofessional learning trajectory would benefit students' practice. A wide range of health and social care teams, including police, practitioners in the statutory sector and voluntary sector of a Sure Start unit, members of a cancer unit and Ear Nose and Throat Team spoke personally about why teamworking is paramount. Evaluations of the DVD showed its potential to align students to their IPE curriculum across ten different professions.

Care is needed in the introduction of an interprofessional curriculum within existing professional education programmes. Poorly presented, this can be badly received and lead to resistance by students. They may vote with their feet and lobby their Heads of Schools serving to send negative messages quickly from year to year. Students will participate in interprofessional learning that is clearly aligned to their learning needs, if they can understand its value to them and their particular practice setting.

Faculty and the wider faculty

The challenges for those in health and social care faculties committed to IPE are well put by Gilbert (2005), when quoting Machievelli, reminds us,

> . . . there is nothing more difficult to take in hand, more perilous to conduct, or more uncertain in its success, than to take the lead in the introduction of a new order of things. Because the innovator has for enemies, all those who have done well under the old conditions, lukewarm defenders in those who may do well under the new.
>
> (Nicolo Machievelli, The Prince, 1513–1516 in Gilbert 2005)

Not only do we need to align language, learning approaches and curriculum timetables but also, and arguably the most challenging, we need to align people. Many education practitioners remain unconvinced, uncertain, ignorant and unwilling to adapt to change or to even consider giving the new curriculum a chance. After all, it wasn't seen as essential in their day. The nature of the facilitative learning required takes many lecturers out of their comfort zone of didactic teaching into the realms of designing and delivering adult learning. Practice educators often remain misinformed about IPE. The disruption of introducing IPE can feel disproportionate and result in a loss of time for students to learn what, the sceptics feel, really matters.

Facilitative team teaching poses resource issues and staff development for this challenging role (Howkins and Bray 2007). The teacher in IPE must be authoritative in their subject and/or its practice, have the ability to recognise the primacy of learning rather than teaching, and enable integration of multiple professional expertises (Anderson *et al.* 2008). Preparation for educators is now seen as vital to the success of any IPE curriculum (Hammick *et al.* 2007). Support to develop these interprofessional facilitation skills is available in the UK through the Centre for the Advancement of Interprofessional Education (www.caipe.org.uk).

Our focus so far has been on what it means for interprofessionalism to be a normative part of health and social care sciences curricula. We finally turn our attention to the process of achieving this.

Mainstreaming the Interprofessional Curriculum: The Process

Experience has taught us that introducing and maintaining an interprofessional curriculum is a journey populated with joy and hazards. The beat of the academic year with systems and processes for introducing change is often the key determinant of the pace of introduction. With novel and contested curriculum changes, this may be at odds with the work of engaging with colleagues in other faculties and institutions. Some ideas fall by the way side in this process; others are swept along not fully developed. Much is gained by the cyclical nature of education, where there is always the next cohort of students to teach and assess, and another opportunity to evaluate the outcomes of interprofessional learning.

Robust evaluation that provides reliable and valid feedback is an essential feature of good educational practice. Nowhere is it more essential than in the early adoption stage of curriculum change. Objective findings from well-planned evaluations are powerful tools in the process of convincing the wider faculty of the need for change. Using the *plan–do–study–act* wheel of reflecting upon individual and collective education practice, again and again, builds experience and expertise and allows well-considered changes to be made to original plans.

It is also good practice to draw upon evidence from systematic reviews (see, for example, Hammick *et al.* 2007) and sound primary studies to inform a particular curriculum development initiative. Responsible interprofessional curriculum planning takes account of some key mechanisms for maximising its positive impact for learners. We have little interest in the simplistic question of whether or not IPE works and would encourage colleagues to respond in a similar vein if asked this question. We do know that finding out what works best, where and for whom in similar contexts can be helpful, in what can be a complex curriculum planning process.

Good intentions and evidence of how to improve the learning and teaching experience are essential, but sometimes not sufficient ingredients to embed change. We believe this to be especially so in relation to changing professional education process. Openness to the ideas and customs of others, an ability to discard treasured ideas and adjust long-held traditional views about what is, and is not, important are equally vital. In Tables 11.2 and 11.3, we use two well-known analytical frameworks (a SWOT and a PESTLE analysis) to identify issues that may arise and demand solutions in the process of embedding IPE in long established programmes tailored to the beliefs and demands of one practitioner group. The tables are populated by the myriad issues that IPE developers may meet. Context will determine what issues are more or less important in your institution. We invite you to adapt each table to your situation as a way of illuminating the key issues that will assist and may impede work on your interprofessional curriculum.

Table 11.2   A SWOT Analysis Related to Developing and Sustaining IPE

Strengths	Weaknesses
• Multiple governmental drivers for learning together to enable better working together in delivery of services to the public • Do we have a choice if curricula are to reflect clinical practice and service delivery? • User-led public service demands joined-up working • Included in professional and statutory body requirements as first post competencies	• Availability of suitable very large and small group learning spaces • Incompatibility of on-campus and in-practice learning timetables • Diverse expectations about teaching and learning styles • Costs of designing new teaching repertoires • Difficulties in easily disaggregating committed funding/resources

Table 11.2 Continued

Opportunities	Threats
• Role of champions • Developing interprofessional leaders • Influence of the students • Sharing of workplace learning spaces by students on different programmes is efficient and sensible • Employability of the newly qualified graduate	• New pressing demands on curriculum • No consensus understanding of the knowledge, skills and attitudes needed for competent interprofessional practice • Change of emphasis and demands by professional bodies • No consensus on how to measure interprofessional competency

Table 11.3 A PESTLE Analysis Related to Developing and Sustaining IPE

Political	Economic
• Role of professional bodies • Conflicting beliefs about the principles of professional education • Not starting with a blank page, impact of tradition and habit/culture	• Can involve long-term need for different physical spaces and potential costly rebuild • Need to put the economic case, consider the positive and negative role of pump priming

Social	Technological
• Teaching about teams is not new in uniprofessional curriculum, but it is different, and this has an impact on some of the subjects in any uniprofessional curriculum, because they have to let go • Risks and benefits to staff and students	• Blended learning opportunities that enable full use of interactive learning systems • e learning opportunities have great appeal to students who are digital natives • The opportunities offered through simulated learning

Legal	Environmental
• Regulatory bodies current power to dictate and whether there maybe future legislation to change professional registration requirements • Ethics: client confidentiality and its impact on interprofessionalism	• Movement of learners between sites • Advantages of virtual interprofessional learning • Need for a sufficiency of practice opportunities for students to develop interprofessional competence

Conclusion

We have argued that improvements in health and well-being services are strongly correlated with ensuring that staff who deliver services experience learning that enables their profession-specific knowledge, skills and attitudes to merge seamlessly with, and carry equal weight to, their interprofessional competence. Along with others, we acknowledge that developing a relevant, effective and efficient interprofessional curriculum, which is accepted as a normal constituent part of professional education, is not easy (Barr and Ross 2006).

Good progress is being made towards sustainability in many places. We offer a summary of what is needed to secure IPE more widely in the future (Box 11.8) and wish you well in sustaining IPE in your context.

Box 11.8 Key Messages for the Practice of Sustaining Interprofessional Education

- Small evaluated pilot initiatives, the development of models that work in the local context, and effective local partnerships.
- A research and evaluation approach and a continuous quality cycle to ensure that the *reformation* and *additions* to the curriculum are evidence-informed and reflect collaborative practice as it happens in practice.
- Robust measurement, through agreed assessment frameworks, of the achievement of interprofessional competence by those engaged in inter-professional learning.
- A student-centred approach to the establishment of interprofessional competencies.
- Theoretically rich curricula design informed by evidence, with a coherent, accepted and long-term resource plan.

Notes

1. *Interprofessional education/training* is those occasions when members (or students) of two or more professions learn with, from and about one another to improve collaboration and the quality of care (CAIPE definition in Hammick *et al.* 2007).
2. The word 'professional' as used here describes a way of behaving rather than particular groups of practitioners.
3. *Curriculum* is an overarching term for all those aspects of education that contribute to the experience of learning: aims, content, mode of delivery, assessment and so on (Freeth *et al.* 2005).

References

Anderson, E. and L. Thorpe. (2008). Early interprofessional interactions: Does student age matter? *Journal of Interprofessional Care* 22 (3), 263–282.

Anderson, E., A. Lennox and S. Petersen. (2003). Learning from Lives – a model for health and social care education in the wider community context. *Medical Education* 37, 59–68.

Anderson, E. and T. Knight. (2003). The three strand model of interprofessional education. *CAIPE Bulletin* (24), Winter 2004, 12.

Barr, H., I. Koppel, S. Reeves, M. Hammick and D. Freeth. (2005). *Effective Interprofessional Education: Argument, Assumption and Evidence.* Oxford: Blackwell Publishing.

Barr, H. and F. Ross. (2006). Mainstreaming interprofessional education in the United Kingdom: A position paper. *Journal of Interprofessional Care* 20 (2), 96–104.

Bernd, D., O. Hans-Uwe and S. Stefan. (2005). New professionalism in social work – A Social Work and Society Series. *Social Work and Society* 3 (2).

Brockopp, D., M. Schooler, D. Welsh, K. Cassidy, P.Y. Ryan, K. Mueggenberg and D.O. Chlebowy. (2003). Sponsored professional seminars: Enhancing professionalism among baccalaureate nursing students. *Journals of Nursing Education* 42 (12), 562–564.

CAIPE Centre for the Advancement of Interprofessional Learning. http://www.caipe.org.uk/ (Accessed 20 May 2009).

Cooper, H., E. Spencer-Dawe and E. McLean. (2005). Beginning the process of teamwork: Design, implementation and evaluation of an inter-professional education intervention for first year undergraduate students. *Journal of Interprofessional Care* 19 (5), 492–508.

Deirdre, C., P.M. Lynch, and R.E. Arnold. (2004). Assessing professionalism; a review of the literature. *Medical Teacher* 26 (4), 366–373.

Department for Education and Skills. (2004). *Children's Trust Pathfinder Projects Grant 2003–04.* London: Stationery Office.

Department of Health. (2001). *NHS Local Improvement Finance Trust (NHS LIFT) Prospectus.* London: Stationery Office.

Department of Health. (2003). *Modernising Medical Careers.* London: HMSO.

Evetts, J. (1999). Professionalisation and professionalism: Issues for interprofessional care. *Journal of Interprofessional Care* 13 (2), 119–128.

Fallsberg, M.B. and M. Hammar. (2000). Strategies and focus at an integrated, interprofessional training ward. *Journal of Interprofessional Care* 14 (4), 337–350.

Fallsberg, M.B. and K. Wijma. (1999). Student attitudes towards the goals of an inter-professional training ward. *Medical Teacher* 21 (6), 576–581.

Freeth, D. (2001). Sustaining interprofessional education. *Journal of Interprofessional Care* 15 (1), 37–46.

Freeth, D., M. Hammick, S. Reeves, I. Koppel and H. Barr. (2005). *Effective Interprofessional Education: Development, Delivery and Evaluation.* Oxford: Blackwell Publishing.

General Medical Council. (1993). *Tomorrow's Doctors: Recommendations on Undergraduate Medical Education.* London: General Medical Council.

General Medical Council. (2003). *Tomorrow's Doctors. Protecting Patients Guiding Doctors. Recommendations on Undergraduate Medical Education.* London: General Medical Council.

Gilbert, J.H.V. (2005). Interprofessional learning and higher education structural barriers. *Journal of Interprofessional Care* 19 (Suppl. 1), 87–106.

Hammick, M., D. Freeth, I. Koppel, S. Reeves and H. Barr. (2007). A best evidence systematic review of interprofessional education BEME Guide No. 9. *Medical Teacher* 29 (8), 735–751 and at http://www.bemecollaboration.org/beme/pages/reviews/hammick.html.

Hean, S., J. MaCleod Clarke, K. Adams and D. Humphries. (2006). Will opposites attract? Similarities and differences in students' perceptions of the stereotype profiles of other health and social care professional groups. *Journal of Interprofessional Care* 20 (2), 162–181.

Hilton, S.R. and H.B. Slotnick. (2005). Proto-professionalism: How professionalisation occurs across the continuum of medical education. *Medical Education* 39, 58–65.

Howkins, E. and J. Bray. (2007). *Preparing for Interprofessional Teaching: Theory and Practice.* Oxford: Radcliffe Publishing.

Jha, V., H.L. Bekker, S.R.G. Duffy and T.E. Roberts. (2007). A systematic review of studies assessing and facilitating attitudes towards professionalism in medicine. *Medical Education* 41, 822–829.

Kennedy report: Learning from Bristol: the report of the public inquiry into children's heart surgery at the Bristol Royal Infirmary 1984–1995: http://www.bristol-inquiry.org.uk/(Accessed 18 August 2008).

Laming Report. (2003). *The Victoria Climbié Inquiry.* Presented to the Secretary of State for Health and the Secretary for the Home Department.

Lennox, A. and E.S. Anderson. (2007). *The Leicester Model of Interprofessional Education: A Practical Guide to Implementation in Health and Social Care Education.* Special Report 9 The Higher Education Academy Subject Centre for Medicine, Dentistry and Veterinary Medicine.

Lennox, A. and S. Petersen. (1998). Development and evaluation of a community based multiagency course for medical students: Descriptive survey. *BMJ* 316, 596–599.

Lennox, A. Beacon Practices. *NHS Beacon Learning Handbook.* Spreading good practice across the NHS 2000/2001, Vol. 1; 238.

Meads, G. and J. Ashcroft. (2005). *The Case for Interprofessional Collaboration in Health and Social Care.* Ed. G. Meads and J. Ashcroft. Oxford: Blackwell Publishing Ltd.

McMenamin, P. (2007). *Body Painting as a Teaching Tool in Teaching Anatomy to Medical Students and Life Drawing Artists.* Trondheim: Association of Medical Education in Europe Conference.

McNair, R.P. (2005). The case for educating health care students in professionalism as the core content of interprofessional education. *Medical Education* 39, 456–464.

Moon, J. (1999). *Reflection in Learning and Professional Development.* London: Kogan Page.

National Health Service. (2000). *NHS Beacons Learning Handbook Vol. 1. Spreading Good Practice Across the NHS.* St Matthews Medical Centre.

National Occupational Standards for Social Work. (2002). Key Role 3. http://www.york.ac.uk/depts/spsw/documents/3SWNOSdocpdffilesedition Apr04.pdf.

NMC. (2007). National Nursing and Midwifery Council: Standards of Proficiency for Pre-registration Nursing Education to Register. Standard 7. http://www.nmc-uk.org/aFrameDisplay.aspx?DocumentID=2616.

Pietroni, R. and C. Pietroni. (1995). *Innovation in Community Care and Primary Health: Marylebone Experiment*. Edinburgh: Churchill Living Stone.

Race, P. (2005). *Making Learning Happen*. London: Sage Publications.

Revans, L. (2002). Victoria Climbié Inquiry. Laming probe reveals scope of communications breakdown. *News Analysis*. Community Care February. www.community-care.co.uk.

Schön, D. (1987). *Educating the Reflective Practitioner*. San Francisco: Jossey Bass.

Smith, R. and E.S. Anderson. (2006). Interprofessional Education. *The Higher Education Academy Social Policy and Social Work*. Report 2: Southampton.

Wackerhausen, S. (2007). *Reflection as Transformation Collaboration and Reflection Across Boundaries*. Krakow: International Conference of the European Interprofessional Network.

Whalley, M. and the Pen Green Centre Team. (2001). *Involving Parents in Their Children's Learning*. London: Sage. www.pengreen.org

Weatherall, D.J. (2006). Science in the undergraduate curriculum during the 20th century. *Medical Education* 40, 195–201.

Wynd, C.A. (2003). Current factors contributing to professionalism in nursing. *Journal of Professional Nursing* 19 (5), 251–261.

Appendix 1

Interprofessional Learning Week

Information Guide for Students

Warwick Medical School, Coventry University and a Primary Care Trust collaborating in interprofessional education

---

Contents

Introduction

Thank you for agreeing to participate

Interprofessional working and education are an essential part of the government's modernisation agenda relating to the pre-registration education of health professionals (Making a Difference [DH 1999], Meeting the Challenge [DH 2000], Learning for Collaborative Practice [DH 2003], Tomorrow's Doctors [GMC 2003]).

It is not a new concept, but has gained prominence in the quest to improve patient care. Working as a team is a central part of patient care and when team members do not communicate it is the patient that reaps the consequences. Coventry University and Warwick Medical School are investigating ways to promote interprofessional education (IPE) in practice to improve the patient's experience within health and social care settings.

CAIPE (The Centre for Advancement of Interprofessional Education) offers the following definition of IPE:

Occasions when two or more professions learn from, with and about each other to improve collaboration and quality of care.

(CAIPE 2002)

The learning week aims to enable pre-registration health professional students to explore the care of ward based patient(s) from a variety of perspectives whilst working with each other to determine the best possible outcomes for such patient(s).

It is important to note that throughout this guide the word 'patient' will be used to describe the individual with a health issue. This in no way fails to recognise that different health and social care professionals use a variety of language to describe the individual. It is an important area to explore when working with other professionals, and also important to recognise that the end goal for all professions is to achieve the best possible outcome for the individual.

Aims and Objectives

Aim

To participate in a multiprofessional group to explore the care of allocated ward based patient(s).

Learning outcomes

By the end of the week, students will be able to:

- Recognise the importance of teamworking to deliver effective patient care
- Begin to compare and contrast the different skills of team members
- Appreciate the importance of placing the ward based patient, and the patient's views at the centre of teamworking
- Actively engage in reviewing the case(s) of an individual ward based patient(s) with members of their own/other profession(s)
- Discuss the patient(s) at a student led multidisciplinary team meeting.

Who Is Involved

This interprofessional learning week is being developed on ward at a local Rehabilitation Hospital with Coventry University and Warwick Medical School. Within the ward the lead professionals from a variety of disciplines that contribute to the ward team will take on an 'expert' role to guide you through the week. The lead expert will be the ward manager who will co-ordinate the week and ensure, in conjunction with the facilitator(s), that you are enabled to meet your objectives for the week.

The lead expert will organise the week in collaboration with the area facilitator(s) (you will meet your facilitators at the beginning of the IPE week). The facilitator(s) will be in daily contact with you, in collaboration with the lead expert. This daily joint contact aims to provide you, as a group, with the opportunity to reflect on your work/findings/thoughts so far in relation to your ward based patient case. The lead expert and the facilitator(s) will encourage you to plan what you hope to achieve before the next meeting.

The Structure of the Week

The timetable will be developed around the individual needs of the ward and the needs of the expert professionals involved. You will have the opportunity to work as a part of a small multiprofessional team in the care of an allocated ward based patient(s). It is anticipated that the patient(s) will be approaching discharge and this will enable you to consider the issues that will face the patient(s) at this time.

The lead expert, following negotiation with the multiprofessional team, will allocate an appropriate ward based patient(s) to your group. Your group will meet on a regular basis throughout the week to work with the patient(s) and to discuss their care. It is anticipated that this will enable you to gain a fuller appreciation of the care provided by different professionals.

You will also have the opportunity to meet with the different experts at the beginning of the week to discuss their role as part of the team, to take part in a multidisciplinary ward round and to discuss your patient(s) at a student led multidisciplinary team meeting at the end of the week.

Experts will also be available during the week to guide you to a greater understanding of their role in the multiprofessional team. It is important that you emerge from the week with an understanding not only of how it feels to work as part of a multiprofessional team, but also of your profession specific role within the team.

You will be given time to gain a greater understanding of working as part of your own professional group, in addition to working as part of a small multiprofessional team.

The Role of the Lead Expert and the Facilitator(s)

The lead expert and the facilitator's roles are key to guiding you so that you, and your group are provided with the opportunity:

- To learn from, with and about each other
- To understand and respect each other's role in your patient(s) case
- To work together as a team
- To maintain, as a team, the focus of patient-centred care

- To discuss each other's roles
- To identify, if and where your roles overlap in the care of your ward based patient(s)
- To identify who will be responsible for the different aspects of care needed by your ward based patient(s).

The Role of the Experts

The range of experts that participate in your experience during the week will differ slightly across the wards. However, the experts will offer a range of experiences for you. The experts, that have a student working within the group, will guide the student throughout the week offering an understanding of the contribution of their profession to multiprofessional working, whilst also ensuring the student's understanding of the unique role of their profession.

The experts, who do not have a student participating but who will be contributing to the week, will ensure that you understand their role in the team. This will be achieved by either discussing their role with you, or by working with your group in the care of your ward based patient(s) during the week.

Time will be allocated on Monday for the experts to discuss their role with you. The experts will also be present at the multidisciplinary meeting towards the end of the week.

Interprofessional student week

Pre-week self-assessment

Which of the following student groups do you belong to? (Tick the appropriate box)

Clinical Psychologist . □   Nurse . . . . □   Radiographer . . . . . . □
Dietitian . . . . □   Occupational Therapist . . □   SALT . . . . □
Doctor . . . . □   Pharmacist . . . . □   Social Worker . . . . . . □
Midwife . . . . □   Physiotherapist . . . . □

Please circle the number relating to your experience or knowledge **prior** to participating in this week.

	poor $\longrightarrow$ excellent				
My understanding of the roles of other health and social care professionals	1	2	3	4	5
My understanding of my own profession's contribution in a team	1	2	3	4	5
My understanding of the role of multidisciplinary meetings in the role of ward based patient care	1	2	3	4	5

My understanding of the impact of interprofessional working on patient/client care	1	2	3	4	5
My understanding of the implications of 'key workers' in patient/client care	1	2	3	4	5
My understanding of how multidisciplinary working will impact on my postgraduate development	1	2	3	4	5

What do you hope to gain from this week?

Please comments on any aspect of the week you would like to see improved

Interprofessional student week

Post-week self-assessment

Which of the following student groups do you belong to? (Tick the appropriate box)

Clinical Psychologist . □   Nurse . . . . □   Radiographer . . . . . . □
Dietitian . . . . □   Occupational Therapist . . □   SALT . . . . □
Doctor . . . . □   Pharmacist . . . . □   Social Worker . . . . . . □
Midwife . . . . □   Physiotherapist . . . . □

Please circle the number relating to your experience or knowledge **after** participating in this week.

	poor	$\longrightarrow$		excellent	
My understanding of the roles of other health and social care professionals	1	2	3	4	5
My understanding of my own profession's contribution in a team	1	2	3	4	5
My understanding of the role of multidisciplinary meetings in the role of ward based patient care	1	2	3	4	5

My understanding of the impact of interprofessional working on patient/client care	1	2	3	4	5
My understanding of the implications of 'key workers' in patient/client care	1	2	3	4	5
My understanding of how multidisciplinary working will impact on my postgraduate development	1	2	3	4	5

Please comment on any aspect of the week you particularly valued

Please comment on any aspect of the week you would like to see improved

Student Timetables

Student multidisciplinary team week

Monday	Tuesday	Wednesday	Thursday	Friday
08.45 Meet ward manager	07.30 Meet on ward. Handover and care for identified patients as a team	Ward round with team	Time for shadowing/ interviews/as you wish	11.30–12.30 Meeting with experts, facilitators and student team to discuss week, ideas about how to improve multidisciplinary team meeting – impact on your patient cases – strengths and areas for improvement in your patient cases.
09.30–11.00 attend multidisciplinary team meeting	Meet facilitators	Meet facilitators	Meet facilitators	Evaluate week
11.00 Meet with facilitators				
LUNCH	LUNCH	LUNCH	LUNCH	LUNCH
Uniprofessional activities	Interview patients	2–3.00 Patient admission procedures with Uniprofession		
	Identify and plan time with agencies			

Facilitator contacts: Andre Bluteau, Ann Jackson, Pat Bluteau

Evaluation Form

Interprofessional Week

State your professional training, e.g. Nurse, Medic	

State year of training	

Please note: 5 is the highest positive response and 1 the lowest indicating a poor outcome

	1	2	3	4	5	
I was **not clear** about what I had to do in this week	1	2	3	4	5	I **was clear** about what I had to do in this week
I **was not looking forward** to working with other undergraduate healthcare professionals	1	2	3	4	5	I **was looking forward** to working with other undergraduate healthcare professionals
The daily facilitation opportunities **were not** supportive	1	2	3	4	5	The daily facilitation opportunities **were** supportive
The patient case study **did not help me** to value the importance of patient centred care in multidisciplinary working	1	2	3	4	5	The patient case study **did help me** to value the importance of patient centred care in multidisciplinary working
The case study **did not help me** to appreciate the range and roles of professionals involved in teamworking in my patient's case	1	2	3	4	5	The case study **did help me** to appreciate the range and roles of professionals involved in teamworking in my patient's case

The format of the case study presentations **was not appropriate**	1	2	3	4	5	The format of the case study presentations **was appropriate**
The mentors **did not** give me sufficient instruction	1	2	3	4	5	The mentors **did** give me sufficient instruction
The information guide **was not** appropriate	1	2	3	4	5	The information guide **was** appropriate
The week **was not** enjoyable	1	2	3	4	5	The week **was** enjoyable
The format of the student led multidisciplinary team meeting **was not** useful	1	2	3	4	5	The format of the student led multidisciplinary team meeting **was** useful
The format of this week **is not worth recommending** to future students	1	2	3	4	5	The format of this week **is worth recommended** to future students

Thank you for taking the time to fill in this evaluation form.

Appendix 2

Interprofessional Learning Week

Information Guide for Experts and Facilitators

Contents

Introduction

Thank you for agreeing to participate in the Interprofessional Week

Interprofessional working and education are an essential part of the government's modernisation agenda relating to the pre-registration education of health professionals (Making a Difference [DH 1999], Meeting the Challenge [DH 2000], Learning for Collaborative Practice [DH 2003], Tomorrow's Doctors [GMC 2003]).

It is not a new concept, but has gained prominence in the quest to improve patient care. Working as a team is a central part of patient care and when team members do not communicate it is the patient that reaps the consequences.

CAIPE (The Centre for Advancement of Interprofessional Education) offers the following definition of IPE:

> Occasions when two or more professions learn from, with and about each other to improve collaboration and quality of care.
>
> (CAIPE 2002)

This learning week aims to enable pre-registration health and social care professional students to explore the care of a ward based patient(s) from a variety of perspectives whilst working with each other to determine the best possible outcomes for the patient(s).

236

It is important to note that throughout this guide the word 'patient' will be used to describe a ward-based individual with a health issue. This in no way fails to recognise that different health and social care professionals use a variety of language to describe the individual. It is an important area to explore when working with other professionals, and also important to recognise that the end goal for all professions is to achieve the best possible outcome for the individual.

Aims and Objectives

Aim

To participate in a multiprofessional group to explore the care of an allocated ward based patient(s).

Learning outcomes

By the end of the week, students will be able to:

- Recognise the importance of teamworking to deliver effective patient care
- Begin to compare and contrast the different skills of team members
- Appreciate the importance of placing a ward based patient, and the patient's views at the centre of teamworking
- Actively engage in reviewing the case of an individual patient with members of their own/other profession(s)
- Discuss the patient(s) at a student led multidisciplinary team meeting.

Who Is Involved

The Stroke unit at a local Rehabilitation Hospital. Within this unit the lead professionals from the variety of disciplines that contribute to the ward team will take on an 'expert' role to guide the students through the week. The lead expert will be the ward manager who will co-ordinate the week and ensure in conjunction with the facilitator(s) that the students are enabled to meet their objectives for the week.

The lead expert will organise the week in collaboration with the area facilitator(s).

The facilitator(s) will be in daily contact with the students in collaboration with the lead expert. The daily joint contact aims to provide the students, as a group, with the opportunity to reflect on their work/findings/thoughts in relation to their patient case. The lead expert and the facilitator(s) will encourage the students to plan what they hope to achieve before the next meeting.

The Structure of the Week

The timetable will be developed according to the individual needs of the unit and the needs of the expert professionals involved. All students will have the opportunity to work as a part of a small multiprofessional team in the care of an allocated ward based patient(s). It is anticipated that the patient(s) will be approaching discharge and this will enable the students to consider the issues that will face the patient(s) at this time.

The lead expert following negotiation with the multiprofessional team will allocate an appropriate ward based patient(s) to the student group. The student group will meet on a regular basis throughout the week to work with the patient(s), and to discuss their care. It is anticipated that this will enable the students to gain a fuller appreciation of the care provided by differing professionals.

Students will also have the opportunity to meet with the different experts at the beginning of the week to discuss their role as part of the team, to take part in a multidisciplinary ward round and to discuss their patient(s) at a student led multidisciplinary team meeting.

Experts will also be available during the week to guide their profession specific student to a greater understanding of their role in the multiprofessional team. It is important that the students emerge from the week with an understanding not only of how it feels to work as part of a multiprofessional team, but also of what their profession specific role was within the team.

Students will be given time to gain a greater understanding of working as part of their own professional group in addition to working as part of a small multiprofessional team.

The Role of the Lead Expert and the Facilitator(s)

The lead expert and the facilitator's roles are key to guiding the students so that they, as a group, are provided with the opportunity:

- To learn from, with and about each other
- To understand and respect each other's role in their ward-based patient(s) case
- To work together as a team
- To maintain, as a team, the focus of patient-centred care
- To discuss each other's roles
- To identify if and where their roles overlap in the care of their patient(s)
- To identify who will be responsible for the different aspects of care needed by their patient(s).

This will be achieved by helping the group to establish ground rules for the week's work, listening to the group's discussion, asking questions, providing ideas, suggesting alternatives and identifying possible resources.

The lead expert and the facilitator(s) should

- Guide the group by, if necessary, initiating and monitoring the activities of each group
- Ensure the group maintains its focus on ensuring delivery of patient-centred and individualised care by assistance, direction, suggestion and intervention where necessary
- Ensure that the students consider their role holistically
- Ensure that each team member has a role and that ground rules are established and adhered to
- Where necessary, suggest areas for further exploration, identify where to access further information or means of accessing relevant professionals
- Assist in developing teamworking and collaboration
- Assist in keeping team members on track during the daily contact
- Ensure that the needs of all participants are met
- Challenge any student assumptions, which may become apparent, especially in relation to different professional roles/stereotypes.

The lead expert will also negotiate with the team and allocate the chosen patient(s) to the students.

The lead expert and the facilitator(s) will also be present at the multidisciplinary meeting, which will be student led.

The Role of the Experts

The experts will offer a range of experiences for the students. The experts that have a student working within the group will guide their student throughout the week offering an understanding of the contribution of their profession to multiprofessional working, whilst also ensuring the student's understanding of the unique role of their profession.

The experts who do not have a student participating but who will be contributing to the week will ensure the student's understanding of their role in the team. This will be achieved by either discussing their role with the students or working with the students in the care of the allocated patient during the pilot week.

Time will be allocated on Monday for the experts to discuss their role with the students. The experts will also be present at the multidisciplinary meeting which will take place at the end of the week.

Appendix 3

Coventry University & University of Warwick

Interprofessional Learning Pathway

Year 1

Contents

Introduction

There is evidence to suggest that when health and social care professionals work together co-operatively, and respect each other's skills, values and knowledge, the result is a more satisfactory, smoother and ultimately less frustrating experience for the patient, client, carer or service user.

But 'interprofessional working' is dependent on individual professionals having a sound understanding of the roles, skills, knowledge and guiding philosophies of other professions. In the Faculty of Health and Life Sciences at Coventry University in collaboration with Warwick Medical School at the University of Warwick, there are 13 separate courses leading to registration as a qualified health and social care professional – and hence a great opportunity to learn with, from and about students from other professions as you proceed through your professional education. Furthermore, the process of discussing your own role and insights with others will, we hope, help you to celebrate the special skills and knowledge that your own profession brings to an integrated model of patient, client, care or service user care.

Through the interprofessional learning pathway at Levels 1, 2 and 3, you will have repeated opportunities to engage with students and qualified professionals to discuss issues and scenarios directly related to patient and client care. These discussions will help you to develop terms of reference and a cognitive framework that will guide you when observing, exploring and reflecting on the multitude of models of multidisciplinary working which you will encounter in practice.

The interprofessional learning pathway is not a module in its own right, though it is linked to a designated module at each level of each course, through its learning outcomes and assessment. We recommend that you take time to thoroughly familiarise yourself with the way in which the interprofessional learning pathway works, and what is expected of you in terms of contribution and assessment.

Aim and Intended Learning Outcomes

Intended learning outcomes (Level 1)

By participating within your virtual learning set (VLS) you should be able to:

1. Explore the range of professions involved in different care or treatment settings and describe aspects of one's own professional role, responsibilities and values to other professionals
2. Utilise communication skills and channels effectively, to share knowledge and ideas in the interprofessional VLS.

Structure and Organisation of the environment

Interprofessional VLS: Year one

At the IPLP launch, you were allocated to an interprofessional student group who will be your 'virtual learning set' for the remainder of the academic year. Each learning set will have an e facilitator (a member of staff or professional practitioner).

The VLS you have been allocated to has its own dedicated discussion space where your deliberations will be visible only to other members of your group and your facilitator.

The first patient/client/service user scenarios will be launched in Blackboard on Monday, Week 1. The story will be revealed in four instalments over four weeks and you will be able to contribute your insights to your group's discussion area, initiating or responding to comments from other students, or to questions from your facilitator.

As the Level 1 interprofessional learning pathway assessment is based around a reflection on a selection of relevant discussion contributions, it is essential that

Instalment	Date
Patient journey launch	Monday, Week 1
Second episode of patient journey	Monday, Week 2
Third episode of patient journey	Monday, Week 3
Fourth episode of patient journey	Monday, Week 4

you log into the IPL pathway web regularly to explore the scenarios and to read, reflect on and contribute to discussion postings.

Accessing VLS

You will be able to access Blackboard from one of the University's (800) open-access computers, or from home and other locations where you may have access to the Internet.

If you are on placement while an online scenario is running, you are expected to continue to login regularly, for example from campus, or from a home connection. It may also be possible to login in from some Trust and Department locations, although these opportunities may be very limited for some types of placement. We hope that the online discussions will be particularly enriched by insights from group members on placement who may be able to relate the discussion to live, current issues they are experiencing.

With your co-operation, we will initiate systems to monitor how and when students on practice placement can access the Internet. This information will be used to build an informal database of (work or community based) Internet access points. It will also be used to formulate safeguards to ensure that students who can demonstrate exceptional difficulties in accessing the Internet on placement are not disadvantaged with regard to assessment.

Requirements of Students

1. *Confidentiality*: In your VLS it is important that you recognise that the content of your discussions is confidential. This is to ensure that students feel that they are working within a safe environment.
2. *Communication*: Your postings to your VLS should be in a manner that demonstrates respect for your colleagues. In order to meet the ILO number 2 it is important that you actively contribute to the activities and discussions on a weekly basis.
3. *Time commitment*: The total *time allocated* for Year 1 is *30 hours*. This includes self-directed time spent reflecting, listening, reading, researching and online time posting messages and participating in discussions.
4. *Frequency on logging in to your VLS*: The very nature of e learning means that participants may log on at any time, day or night. This means that you will find that some of your colleagues may have left messages and answered questions before you have even read the original question. A good mechanism

for dealing with this to log on little and often – in this way you read messages as they arrive sequentially, provides you with time to think before posting and ensures that the volume of messages is not overwhelming – remember there may be up to 14 other colleagues in your set which could amount to a considerable number of postings.

5. *Ground rules*: Potential ground rules within the VLS were discussed at the launch of the IPLP. These will be revisited in week 1 to enable negotiation within the whole group and to ensure that all members are agreed on the final rules.

Frequently Asked Question

I cannot log on

Email your facilitator – you will find your *facilitator's email address at the end* of this book. Keep trying to log on at various intervals. Your email will be logged and reported to the IT support team on the IPLP. *It is very important that you do make contact as failure to do so will not be considered a reason for non-participation.*

How do I contact my facilitator?

You will find you facilitator's email address at the back of this book and online in your VLS. Spend time exploring this new environment to become familiar with how it works and its layout. Email your facilitator and colleagues if you are unsure about anything – it is likely that many of your colleagues are also feeling the same way.

Can we meet up as a group?

Yes, you are welcome to meet as a group but you will need to organise this yourselves. Remember that many of you will be out on placements and this may be some distance away, so please think carefully when, and if you decide to this, so that it is inclusive to all.

I need advice about the assessment

There is information and guidelines on the Blackboard site about the assessment. If you still have unanswered questions or queries concerning the assessment, you should contact your facilitator and he/she will be able to answer them.

Can I chat online?

Yes, there are facilities online to allow this. It works in the same way as any normal chat line. The best way to learn how to use this to experiment. You will be able to see if any of your colleagues are online so you can send an invitation to chat. Your facilitator will be able to help you should you experience any problems.

I am out on placement and cannot find a computer with online access?

Please report this as soon as possible to your facilitator. If you are unable to contact your facilitators, if there is no email access, please phone the nominated leads at your university. Your message will then be passed onto your facilitator.

I am ill

You must inform your facilitator that you are unwell and therefore unable to take part in that week's activity and discussion. All sickness will be monitored and you should follow the normal sickness policy for your professional course.

I need an extension – whom do I contact?

The standard university guidelines for extensions should be followed. Your facilitator will be the person you need to contact for an extension.

What happens if I am referred on this module?

If you are referred on this module, you will receive written feedback on your reflective wrapper outlining areas for improvement. You will be expected to re-submit your work following consultation with your marking team (they will be identified on your feedback).

I am really struggling with learning online?

Initially, if you are new to this learning environment, it will feel very strange. Email your facilitator and explain your anxieties – such feelings are not uncommon – your facilitator will be ready and able to support you.

IPLP Year 1 Assessment Guidelines

Coursework Assessment Task

A selection of online, interprofessional discussion contributions with a 500-word reflective wrapper.

IP learning outcomes

- Explore the range of professions involved in different care or treatment settings and describe aspects of one's own professional role, responsibilities and values to other professionals.
- Utilise communication skills and channels effectively to share knowledge and ideas in the interprofessional group.

Guidelines for the coursework

In order to successfully complete the coursework, you must hand in a *500 word Reflective Wrapper* (see Activity Three) *as well as an Appendix* showing evidence of contribution to the Discussion Forum (see Activities One and Two).

Activity One – Contribute to the Discussion Forum

During the lifetime of the scenario, you must regularly read and contribute to your group's online discussion in order to produce evidence that you have contributed to it.

Activity Two – Produce evidence of contribution to the online discussion as an Appendix

Select a minimum of 3 (maximum 6) contributions that *you* have made to your Discussion Forum in which you have felt you have meaningfully* attempted to explain aspects of the role, responsibilities, knowledge and values of your own profession to students of other professions (in the context of the patient/client scenario which your group has discussed).

In addition, select a minimum of 3 (maximum 6) contributions from other group members which can be used to illustrate some of your reflections (see below).

Compile and download the contributions for printing as an Appendix to your 'Reflective Wrapper' (see *Technical Tips* below).

Activity Three – write a 500-word Reflective Wrapper

In this 'wrapper' you should address two issues (either sequentially or in an integrated manner) and you can decide how much of the word count to devote to each issue.

First, you should compose a brief summary of your understanding of the role of *your own* profession in the scenario (as represented by yourself and other group members through the online discussion). Be sure to state which scenario you are referring to at the top of the reflective summary and, where appropriate, cross reference your summary to relevant discussion contributions in your Appendix.

Second, compose a personal reflection on some of the things you have learned about professional roles through engagement with the patient/client scenario and relevant online discussion.

Where appropriate, cross reference your reflections to relevant discussion contributions in the Appendix (e.g. 'Discussion Postings X and Y reflect some of the differences in opinion our group had re which professional group had most contact with the patient').

---

*Meaningful contributions should show evidence of original thought (either as a query or as response to someone else's query). It does not include minor responses such as 'I agree'.

When composing your reflection, you may find it useful to use the following questions to guide your commentary:

- What aspects of my professional role, responsibilities and values was I able to share with my group?
- What knowledge did I draw on (lectures, experience, asking a professional etc.)
- What new knowledge did I learn about the roles of other professions?
- Has my perception of the roles, responsibilities and values of my own and other professions been altered in any way?

Technical Tips for Selecting and Printing Discussion Postings

- You may find it helpful to select the **✎ Discussions** icon in the left-hand toolbar in Blackboard. You can then select **All Topics** or **All my posts**
- Select messages you want to save or print by clicking in the empty box to the left of the Subject Heading □ ⊞ **Activity 1.2** (If there are more than ten messages in the discussion thread, you will have to display the rest of the messages by selecting the message numbers from the drop down box then clicking the green arrowhead to the right of the box.

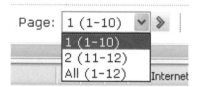

- When you have selected the messages, click the **Create Printable View** button, then **Print**.
- Alternatively, display the posting(s) you want to print on the screen, highlight the posting with the mouse and press **Ctrl-C** to copy. Open a Word document, then press **Ctrl-V** (Paste) to paste it into the Word document. In this way you can build up a selection of potential postings to **Save** and/or **Print**.

Assignments should be handed in online via a *drop box* which is situated in the IPLP Blackboard. If you experience problems finding this box, please contact your facilitator. Further details will also be found on the WebCT site.

SUBMISSION DATE:

Evaluation

We will be asking you to evaluate the experience of the IPLP after you have undertaken the work and your assignment. Pat Bluteau and Ann Jackson will be co-ordinating this.

Facilitator's Email addresses

Appendix 4

Coventry University & University of Warwick

Interprofessional Learning Pathway

Facilitator Guide: Year 3

Contents

Introduction

There is an increasing body of evidence to support the view that learning with, from and about each other during professional training leads to enhanced capacity for teamwork and partnership working (Freeth et al., 2002) – cornerstones of recent Health and Social Care Reforms in the UK. These reforms include increased flexibility of service provision (as embodied in National Service Frameworks) as well as commitment to avoid the 'communication failures' at the heart of notable failures highlighted by the Victoria Climbie, Bristol Heart Surgery, and Harold Shipman enquiries.

Respect for, and knowledge of the roles of other health and social care professionals is also likely to lead to better and more consistent information for the patient, client, service user or carer – an issue which has been consistently highlighted when the views of patients, clients, service users and carers have been sought.

Evidence also suggests that when health and social care professionals work together co-operatively, and respect each others skills, values and knowledge, the result is a more satisfactory, smoother, and ultimately a less frustrating experience for the patient, client, carer or service user.

But 'interprofessional working' is dependent on individual professionals having a sound understanding of the roles, skills, knowledge and guiding philosophies of other professions. In the Faculty of Health and Life Sciences at Coventry University in collaboration with Warwick Medical School at the University of Warwick, there are 14 separate courses leading to registration as a qualified health and social care professional – and hence a great opportunity to learn with, from and about students from other professions as they proceed through their professional education. Furthermore, through the process of discussing their own role and insights with others, the students will, we hope, celebrate the special skills and knowledge that their own profession brings to an integrated model of patient, client, carer or service user care.

Through the IPLP at Levels 1, 2 and 3, students will have repeated opportunities to engage with other students and qualified professionals to discuss issues and scenarios directly related to patient and client care. These discussions will help them to develop terms of reference and a cognitive framework that will guide them when observing, exploring and reflecting on the multitude of models of multidisciplinary working which they will encounter in practice.

The IPLP is not a module in its own right, though it is linked to a designated module at each level of each course through its learning outcomes and assessment.

Educational Rationale for the Interprofessional Learning Pathway (IPLP)

The aim of the strategy for the curriculum in relation to the IPLP is:

> *To enable students to explore issues related to achieving effective and appropriate interprofessional working in practice in order to improve the quality of care for patients and/or clients*

In order to achieve this aim, interprofessional learning outcomes (IPLOs) are contained in each course every year. You will be facilitating students to address three IPLOs. For year three these outcomes are:

1. Critically analyse how knowledge of your own and other professionals' roles impact on patient care.
2. Identify opportunities for integrated assessment/care planning and critically evaluate their impact on the patient/client/carer/service user.
3. Critically analyse examples of good practice in multidisciplinary practice settings.

Structure and Organisation of the Environment

Interprofessional Virtual Learning Sets: Year Three

Students are allocated to an interprofessional student group which will be their 'virtual learning set' (VLS, also called 'discussion group'), for the duration of year three IPLP. Each VLS has between 13–15 students. As a facilitator, you will have 1 or 2 VLS, both groups will be studying the same scenario but both VLS will work independently of each other.

The time allocated to facilitate the VLS sets in Year 3 is 10 hours per group. This includes the time spent on facilitation online activity and online marking over the four-week period.

Your role as a facilitator this year will be:

- To encourage participation in online activities and facilitate online discussion around the scenarios and to mark the students online discussions.
- To contact students with formative feedback regarding their progress in the assessment task by the end of the second week.
- To email any missing students by the beginning of the second week, and if they do not respond, to email the professional lead with the name of the missing student by the end of week 2.
- To copy Pat Bluteau and Learning Technologist into emails concerning missing students.

During the online delivery of the IPLP you have access to a facilitator support area on which you will find an overview of the IPLP scenario. The scenarios will be released in weekly instalments.

Each VLS has been allocated its own dedicated discussion space where student deliberations will be visible only to the student group and to you as the facilitator.

The first scenarios will be launched in CUOnline on . . . . The scenarios will be revealed in four instalments over four weeks:

Instalment	Date
Journey launch	Monday Week 1
Second episode of patient journey	Monday Week 2
Third episode of patient journey	Monday Week 3
Fourth episode of patient journey	Monday Week 4

Each instalment will be released by 12 noon on Monday of that week.

Accessing Virtual Learning Sets

The students will be able to access CUOnline from the University's open-access computers, or from home, placements, libraries or internet cafes and other locations where they may have access to the Internet.

It is essential that facilitators are familiar with the login process before the start of the scenario. Voluntary remedial CUOnline access workshops are available to students and facilitators – by contacting the Learning Technologist on . . . . or emailing him on . . . .

Full guidance on how to access CUOnline is available from the leaning technologist in a separate guide.

Requirements of Students

1. **Read ALL information given in hardcopy and online**: Remember to familiarise yourself with the information in this handbook. Further information will be made available on the IPLP web itself, including notes and guidelines regarding the assignment. Hints and tips are often given using the CUOnline pop up 'Announcement' facility (turn-off any pop up blockers when using CUOnline). When online delivery gets underway your facilitator may give specific instructions about which discussion threads to use to post your responses to the e-activities. There will also be an area on the site for you to post additional queries and questions about technical aspects of the site.

2. **Confidentiality**: In your VLS it is important that you recognise that the content of your discussions is confidential. This is to ensure that students feel that they are working within a safe environment. As needs arise, access to the boards may be given to other staff at the discretion of the IPLP project team.

3. **Communication**: Your postings to your VLS should be in a manner that demonstrates respect for your colleagues. In order to meet the intended learning outcomes it is important that you actively contribute to the activities and discussions on a weekly basis. If you do not engage in your group's discussion you will not pass the IPLP strand.

4. **Time Commitment**: The total **time students are allocated** for Year 3 is *60 hours*. This includes self-directed time spent reflecting, listening, reading, researching and online time posting messages and participating in discussions.

5. **Frequency on logging in to your VLS**: The very nature of e learning means that participants may log on at any time of day or night. This means that you will find that some of your colleagues may have left messages and answered questions before you have even read the original question. A good mechanism for dealing with this is to **log on little and often** – in this way you read messages as they arrive sequentially, to provide you with time to think before posting and ensures that the volume of messages is **not overwhelming** – remember there may be up to 14 or more other colleagues in your set which could amount to a considerable number of postings.

6. **Ground Rules**: Potential ground rules within the VLS were discussed in years 1 and 2 of the IPLP strand. As Year 3 students you are expected to observe ground rules at all times.

7. **Plagiarism**: You must ensure that your posts are in your own original words, and an honest account of your own thoughts; not just a straight copy of what a colleague has written. Where you are citing or quoting someone else you

must make this clear; (use 'quotation marks' or *italics*, for instance). One of the best ways to avoid suspicions of plagiarism is to post your work early, and regularly, and not leave everything to the last few days, when it is harder to be original.

Requirements of Facilitators

1. **Leave:** Facilitation has been shown to play a key role in the success and continuity of student involvement in the online learning. Without frequent facilitation input postings from group members diminishes, and the group 'dies'. It is important then that facilitators who have any kind of leave booked for the duration of the online learning and/or the launch should arrange for cover from other members of their professional group. Similarly any kind of ongoing unpredicted leave such as sickness should be covered. Please inform both Pat Bluteau, and the IPLP professional co-ordinator of any annual leave, and the name of person covering your absence, which has been agreed by your line manager.
2. Log into CUOnline and provide an online presence to discussion group(s) at least two times per week.
3. Use the designated IPLP Facilitator's area as a first port-of-call for any queries, concerns or suggestions about the IPLP online delivery. Contact non-participating students by the beginning of week 2 and encourage them to participate, reminding them of the assessment requirements of Year 3 IPLP.
4. Inform the professional lead with details of any non-participating student by the end of week two.
5. **Accessing CUOnline:** CUOnline has specific browser requirements and it is likely that some students may experience problems accessing the environment because of outdated browsers. Advice on overcoming this problem can be found in the IT information accompanying this document. It is important that as a facilitator you log information from all students experiencing difficulties. IT staff will need to know the location and access point. Students should be encouraged to log in at the internet cafes or within libraries where the browsers will be up to date and accessing CUOnline should not be a problem.
6. **Log in User name:** Students and facilitators should log into the CUOnline using the accompanying guidelines. Your university user name and password should be used to log in.
7. **Log in Problems:** All students are asked to check whether they can access the web site during the weeks prior to the start of the online learning so that access difficulties can be identified and dealt with (if possible). Students experiencing difficulty will contact their facilitator who should notify details to the Learning Technologist.
8. **Facilitator Support:** An online meeting place, CUOnline web, of all facilitators will be identified and available for facilitators to obtain any support or answer queries whilst the VLS are active; the full details of the scenario will

be made available to facilitators. Facilitators can also access their professional IP co-ordinator (see below) and Pat Bluteau.

9. During the IPLP delivery, mark the Students postings, and return (by email) the marking grid to Pat Bluteau with a list of the marks from each group by the agreed deadline (see assessment flowchart).
10. Participate in the overall evaluation of the IPLP by completing the Facilitator's Evaluation Questionnaire which is made available in the Facilitator's area towards the end of the online period.
11. Post a welcome message and set up threads prior to the start of each week (example welcome messages and posts can be found on facilitator web).

Professional Co-ordinators

Essentially, the role of the professional co-ordinator is to co-ordinate the teaching and particularly the assessment of students within their discipline at second and third attempt. Facilitators should liaise with their relevant professional co-ordinator regarding:

- Any professional issue which affects IPLP.
- Any planned or unplanned leave which affects their ability to meet the requirements of an IPLP facilitator.
- Students who are not participating by the end of week 2.

The professional co-ordinators are:

Profession	Name	Email
Adult Nursing		
Children's nursing		
Dietetics		
Learning Disability		
Medicine		
Mental Health Nursing		
Midwifery		
Occupational Therapy		
Physiotherapy		
Social Work		

Assessment Information

Coursework Assessment Task

Online interprofessional discussion contributions.

IPLP learning outcomes

- Critically analyse how knowledge of your own and other professionals' roles impact on patient care.
- Identify opportunities for integrated assessment/care planning and critically evaluate their impact on the patient/client.
- Critically analyse examples of good practice in multidisciplinary practice settings.

Guidelines for the Coursework

In order to successfully complete the coursework and demonstrate that you have met the Year 3 IPLP learning outcomes, you must contribute postings online and complete all of the e-activities. This is very important as it is your contributions online which will be assessed.

N.B. If your contributions are *unsatisfactory* and you are referred or deemed unsatisfactory at the first attempt you will be required to submit a 1200-word reflection which will offer a critique of your postings in relation to the non-achievement of the learning outcomes.

In order to successfully complete Level 3 IPLP, you must:

- Regularly read and contribute to your group's online discussion in order to produce evidence that you have contributed to them.
- Complete the e-activities which demonstrate engagement with your online colleagues.
- Include in your online postings reflections on the scenario, and from your practice experiences.
- Respond to the contribution of others.
- Elements of your postings should show critical analysis and evaluation.
- Reference only when you are directing colleagues to further information, the emphasis of your discussion should be focussed on meaningful engagement within the group.

It might help you to consider some of the following questions when you draw on examples from practice:

- How do your own and other professionals assess patients? What are the differences between the assessments?
- How much responsibility does each profession take for a particular aspect of patient care, for example, diagnosis, wound care, prescribing treatment?
- What are the challenges that different professionals face?
- Which aspects of care do the different professionals lead on?

Submitting the Assignment

The assessment for the IPLP will relate to the contributions that you have made during the four week online discussion period. Your facilitator will mark your work online. To allow for issues beyond the control of either yourself or the IPLP team you will be allowed to continue posting for one week after the groups have completed, if for any reason you have been unable to complete your final postings by the............, however the group will not be facilitated during the period from the.................., but facilitators will take these postings into account when marking your work.

FINAL POSTING DATE:............- **In order to pass students are required to meaningfully complete 80% of e-activities.**

Marking Process

The assessment for the IPLP will relate to the contributions the student has made during the four week online discussion period. You will mark their work online. To allow for issues beyond the students or the IPLP team's control they will be allowed to continue posting for one week after the groups have completed if for any reason you have been unable to complete your final postings by the........., however the group will not be facilitated during the period from the...................., but facilitators will take these postings into account when marking students work.

COMPLETED MARKING TO PAT BLUTEAU:

Assessment Grid:

Interprofessional Learning Pathway. Year 3		
STUDENT: FACILITATOR PROFESSIONAL GROUP MODERATOR	MODULE: DATE:	
IPLP Learning outcomes to be demonstrated within the assignment Students should: 1. Critically analyse how knowledge of your own and other professionals' roles impact on patient care. 2. Identify opportunities for integrated assessment/care planning and critically evaluate their impact on the patient/client. 3. Critically analyse examples of good practice in multidisciplinary practice settings.		
In order to achieve a pass students are required to **meaningfully complete 80% of e-activities;**		
Contribute postings that demonstrate engagement in the content of the learning resource and the related activities.		

Contribute an appropriate number of respectful meaningful postings with minimal prompting to facilitate group discussion.		
Contribute postings that contain elements of critical analysis and evaluation relevant to your own and other group members contributions.		
Contribute postings that contain examples from practice which both illuminate best practice and draw on examples where improvements were necessary.		
Comments		

Evaluation

We will be asking both students and facilitators to evaluate the experience of the IPLP. During the last week of the online delivery the student evaluation questionnaire will be accessible via the IPLP web. The facilitator evaluation will be available via the facilitator support area. Evaluations are used to inform the development of IPLP and the evaluation process is managed by Pat Bluteau (CIPeL) and Ann Jackson (Warwick University).

Index

The lesson plan lan proposing to do here.